HEALTH POLICY
FOR HEALTH CARE
PROFESSIONALS

HEALTH POLICY
FOR HEALTH CARE PROFESSIONALS

PETER L. BRADSHAW AND GWENDOLEN BRADSHAW

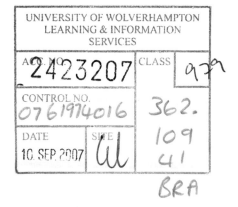
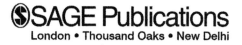

SAGE Publications
London • Thousand Oaks • New Delhi

First published 2004

 SAGE Publications Ltd
1 Oliver's Yard
55 City Road
London EC1Y 1SP

SAGE Publications Inc.
2455 Teller Road
Thousand Oaks, California 91320

SAGE Publications India Pvt Ltd
B-42, Panchsheel Enclave
Post Box 4109
New Delhi 110 017

British Library Cataloguing in Publication data

A catalogue record for this book is available from
the British Library

ISBN 0 7619 7400 8
ISBN 0 7619 7401 6 (pbk)

Library of Congress Control Number: 2004094409

Typeset by C&M Digitals (P) Ltd., Chennai, India
Printed and bound in Great Britain by Athenaeum Press, Gateshead

CONTENTS

HEALTH POLICY: A COMMENTARY FOR HEALTH PROFESSIONALS

INTRODUCTION

This book has been written for health service practitioners and other students of health policy. It assumes some basic understandings of the subject that it intends to enhance by extending the capacity of the reader to assess and analyse the current workings of health services in Britain, especially in relation to the National Health Service (NHS) and the caring agencies with which it works. The text seeks to illuminate the options for action that are available to governments and it draws attention to the slippery nature of health policy and provides conformation that there is no 'right way' to proceed for those who make policy decisions. Someone else, and by no means only in an opposing political party, can usually think of a better way to do things!

The text approaches its task by raising awareness of major themes within health policy that are both current and enduring and will remain so irrespective of the political persuasion of the government that is in office. The book will thus assist practitioners with the interpretation of policy and provide explanations for its implementation at the level at which they function.

The work begins from the premise that a persistent conflict exists within the construction and implementation of health policy. This involves the central concern of strategy makers at government level to act for the collective good that frequently creates tension for managers and for practitioners trying to align services with individual patient need and choice. Health care and the policies that govern it are a very public matter, yet simultaneously an individual and personal one. So while policy intends to be therapeutic, it can also be stressful for those who put it into practice.

This raises debates about the central principles on which the NHS was founded to which successive governments have subscribed. These concern the fundamental constituents of social justice that provide the ethos in which practitioners work to deliver services to patients and it is these elements that the book will investigate. It will therefore:

- locate health policy within the broader ideological framework of welfare state provision;
- examine in detail the nature of health policy in the life of recent governments and scrutinise the feasibility of achieving the current objectives set for the NHS;
- scrutinise the more difficult obstacles to modernisation;
- evaluate critically the funding mechanisms for health care in Britain and consider the alternatives available to governments to pay for it;
- appraise the dynamics of power and control within the NHS;
- identify issues for health policy in the next decade.

The work is based on these six seemingly discrete themes but the reader will quickly conclude that they interconnect and inform each other and act as pieces in a jigsaw that accumulate as the puzzle is built up. Relevant policy documents, their principles and critiques of them are quoted from a diverse range of sources from government documents through to its most trenchant critics, and a detailed bibliography is cited to enable readers to further pursue topics of personal interest.

The book will thus differ from its comparators in its focus. While it will not avoid key features of government strategy it will consistently encourage consideration of these in terms of local circumstances that affect those on the front line who provide direct services to patients.

Chapter 1 will identify the prelude to today's health services through an examination of the ideological, political and economic context for the public services in Britain. It will thus consider those significant precursor events that shaped the environment in which the present-day NHS exists. In doing so, the chapter will also locate the NHS within the overall provision of public services for the nation.

In the second chapter the modernisation agenda for the NHS will be scrutinised. Its coverage will build on the factors identified in Chapter 1. In particular it will address the prolific modernisation plans that were commenced following the election of New Labour in 1997. This state of flux will continue relentlessly for the foreseeable future irrespective of which government is in office because of its magnitude, its irreversible nature and because all the major parties are committed to their own version of health service reform.

Chapter 3 examines the major challenges for a modernised NHS. Despite its claims about modernisation, the *NHS Plan* can be seen as sustaining, through improved capability and additional assets, the old NHS model that is dominated by the provision of acute care (DOH, 2000a). Its targets therefore have a flavour of political pragmatism about them, notably in their pressure to get results rapidly. The *Plan* contains much that is well intended. But for its successful implementation, several major key factors will receive careful consideration. These are: the decentralisation of authority and the creation of genuinely localised health services; the leadership conundrum in health services; the patient as a consumer; and, lastly, patient choice and the role of competition.

Reference is made throughout the book to the equity principles on which the NHS was founded and to the ways in which governments adhere to these. It is these objectives concerning fairness within the NHS that also form the kernel of the debate about how it should be funded. Chapter 4 deals therefore with the generation of funding and appraises alternative ways to pay for health care that is the root cause of so much controversy about its future. All governments recognise tacitly that meeting all of the ambitious objectives set in 1948 all of the time is unachievable in practice and creates the funding problems of the NHS that confront any political administration, chancellor of the exchequer or secretary of state for health.

The NHS is an esteemed institution despite any critics it may have and this adds to its intense politicisation. Chapter 5 will analyse the organisation, direction and control of the service that have proven so elusive to secure throughout its history. Ultimately the secretary of state for health is in charge of the NHS. Through the Civil Service and the Department of Health and its subordinate agencies, government policy is designed to be cascaded in a linear fashion through the various levels of the service to be translated into practical action wherever patients are treated. A feature of New Labour, however, has been the influence on policy that has been exerted by sources outside the Civil Service by academic theorists, special advisers and, by no means least, the party's media managers (Hunter, 2002). The chapter will consider selectively the relative contribution of the major aspects of power and control that will include the macro-management of the NHS and its regulation, the micro-management of the NHS and its organisational context, the power of the medical profession and the relationship between doctors and managers.

The concluding chapter will consider the shorter-term future for the NHS and for health policy by returning to consider more fully some themes that were introduced earlier. These will include the target culture, foundation hospitals, payment by results, patient choice and the Patient's

Passport. The text will then proceed to provide a broader account of the options that might arise to provide health care in general as the decade progresses by examining the challenges for the public health through those predictable factors such as an ageing population and the growth of new technology. It will also scrutinise radical policy options that might be employed to confront these. The book will conclude that during its illustrious history the NHS has often lacked a clear philosophy and rationale, hence its purpose has lacked clarity. Medical technology has appealed to the masses and has led the direction of the service irrespective of its cost or its efficacy. The modern New Labour era has seen a transformation that, although heavy-handed in some respects, has created a new decisive direction and purpose for the NHS that goes some way in confronting reality head-on.

Health service professionals operate on a need-to-know basis and are experts in seeing the fine detail in the way things are running on the front line. This work offers them a chance to view the bigger screen that often they do not have time to contemplate. It does this by the careful selection of a set of external reference points that enable an investigation of the service to occur by exposing those more subtle leavers that have purchase on the professional lives of all health service staff. It therefore provides compelling reading for anyone who wants to navigate a way through these complex debates.

ONE

THE PRELUDE TO TODAY'S NATIONAL HEALTH SERVICE
THE IDEOLOGICAL, POLITICAL AND ECONOMIC CONTEXT FOR THE PUBLIC SERVICES IN BRITAIN

This chapter will examine those significant precursor events that shaped the environment in which the present-day NHS exists. In doing so, this will also locate the NHS within the overall provision of public services for the nation.

THE REASONS FOR THE WELFARE STATE IN BRITAIN, 1948–70

Any attempts to study the workings of the welfare state require careful consideration of its history as well as a rigorous analysis of its strengths and weaknesses. The welfare state in Britain, of which the NHS is a major and enduring part, is complex. It originates from the Beveridge Report, which was the major plank of post-World War II social reconstruction (HMSO, 1942). The report provided a set of welfare principles for improved social justice for British citizens. It thus paved the way for a legislative framework to tackle five areas of serious need that the report had identified (Timmins, 1996). These were:

- want;
- disease;
- ignorance;
- squalor;
- idleness.

In embarking on this ambitious task the first post-war Labour government assumed full state responsibility for vast areas of human well-being. It did this in the ideological belief that market competition could not deliver services for people and meet vital areas of human need. The market economy had failed the population in the inter-war years when much of it experienced unemployment, poverty, poor educational standards, poor health and poor housing. Market forces had failed to supply these important social goods and to deliver essential services. The government thus felt that large-scale, collectivist state intervention was required to meet this unmet need and that only this mechanism could effectively and fairly deliver the volume and quality of services that were required by the post-war population. Its doctrine rejected the market system that had preceded World War II as morally divisive because of its emphasis on the individual and especially on individual acquisitiveness. Total reliance on market exchange as the basis for providing welfare had produced a nation that was socially divided through the unfair way in which it distributed opportunities to its people.

These early social policies on the relief of need were based on citizenship theory (Titmuss and Morris, 1973, 1976; Andrews, 1991). This argues that although at a fundamental level the welfare state provides a necessary safety net, it is also a desirable thing for moral reasons. This line of thinking contends that the welfare state:

- relieves the effects of poverty and other dire forms of social need and protects the most vulnerable people in society;
- lessens social inequality through redistribution of the national wealth from those who have a comfortable standard of living to those who have not;
- promotes an ethically conscious society in which citizens are prepared to contribute willingly through various forms of taxation towards services that they do not often use themselves;
- contributes to the development of individual character and makes each person a more responsible citizen;
- lays the foundation for shared beliefs and values that strengthens communities through a common morality and a consensus on what is right and what is wrong.

The welfare state is a by-product of a strong economy and of economic growth. In order to achieve its ambitious social policy intentions the 1945 Labour government needed an economic policy that would make its plans affordable. The natural ally to Beveridge's welfare policy was the economic theory of John Maynard Keynes (Keynes, 1973; Stewart, 1993). This theory provided a stark contrast to the economic thinking that had preceded it. Keynes's ideas provided a replacement strategy for a system that stemmed from the late 18th century that had its origins in the work of Adam Smith (Fry, 1992).

Smith's principles had thus been the predominant determinant of economic activity for over 250 years. These principles adhere unswervingly to free markets where a system of exchange (based on the price mechanism) distributes all goods and services, including those public services that the welfare state was intending to provide. The doctrine supports a view that the individual is paramount in the process of exchange that is based on vigorous competition. An underlying assumption of this market economic theory is that state interference in the economy is inferior to letting individuals make economic judgements for themselves. Within this thinking, individuals are believed to be naturally selfish, and it is only by encouraging them to operate out of personal self-interest that they will optimise their personal gain from any transactions in which they are involved. Competition, therefore, is the major motivator of rational economic behaviour within this system of market exchange and it is believed that its efficiency stems firstly from its capacity to reward the most successful who survive and prosper and, secondly, because it also forces the weakest and most inefficient competitors to go out of business.

The policies originating from Beveridge's view of the world clearly needed to radically modify this former free-market orientation. What Keynes advocated to afford his bold macro-economic plan for welfare reform required unprecedented state intervention in the management of the economy. This economic plan ran in parallel to the way the state intended to intervene so extensively to provide new types of public services. Put simply, Keynesian economics ensured that:

- State intervention in the economy secured full employment.
- The government had to intervene to control interest rates, taxation policy and public spending.
- The government had a responsibility to stimulate economic growth and to control and create jobs. In practice, this was achieved by substantial state ownership of most major industries.
- The outcome was improved productivity, increased exports and better wages for more people with an overall redistribution of wealth amongst the population.

This way of managing the economy gave way to post-war regeneration and an exponential improvement in living standards for the people. Throughout the 1950s and 1960s both Conservative and Labour governments remained committed both to Keynesian economics and to the expansion of the public services, and all of this was possible because of the strong economy that was both generated and sustained. The population thus experienced a generalised prosperity and had access to a new range of consumer goods and saw no reason to change. The vast majority of British people became better fed, better housed, had better hospitals and schools, and enjoyed benefits that they had never formerly contemplated.

THE 1970S AND ORIGINS OF DISSENT ABOUT THE BRITISH PUBLIC SERVICES

While the British economy remained relatively strong, all shades of political opinion were totally committed to a welfare state that was fuelled by these Keynesian economic policies. But the 1970s were to see a dramatic change in attitude towards both the economy and, more especially, towards public expenditure and the way in which public services were funded. Periods of alternating inflation and economic stagnation began to take their toll politically. During inflationary times, goods became more expensive and were less affordable at home and were more difficult to export. For the first time in post-war Britain, economic recession began to be experienced and the economy became stagnant, economic resources to pay for the public services were scarce and this resulted in service shortages. All of this was compounded by the rising expectations of an electorate that had become accustomed to nothing other than growing and improving levels of public services.

The Labour and Conservative governments that ruled during the 1970s were frequently under pressure from the trade unions for demands for better wages and improved working conditions. Both governments therefore were pressurised into promises that they could not keep. Neither they nor employers succeeded in managing the coercion from trade unions. These powerful organisations used their bargaining power in the public and private sectors of the economy and made wage claims that the economy just could not sustain. The economic triumphs of the 1950s and 1960s were thus succeeded by steep economic decline in the British economy (Johnson, 1991).

By the 1970s the state also found itself in possession of a range of public services that over a 30-year period had become increasingly extensive and sophisticated. At the foundation of the welfare state it had been intended to provide public services to meet a range of basic human needs. But these service organisations such as the NHS had burgeoned into massive, almost monopolistic, institutions that began to provide far more extensively than had been envisaged. The remit for services thus extended beyond meeting basic needs to catering for the complex personalised requirements of the population. Therefore, it was only when the economy became unable to pay adequately for this plethora of public service institutions that a new powerful debate about them began. The arguments that emerged were based on two principal propositions that concerned the entire intellectual rationale for the welfare system. These included:

- The ideological beliefs that the welfare state was devised for a former era and that its services were irrelevant to a modern capitalist economy and therefore needed a drastic overhaul.
- Economic arguments to accompany this dogma that suggested that Keynesian economics had not managed to halt Britain's economic decline and were in similar need of refurbishment.

Much of this new debate emanated from the opinions of what was to become known as the 'New Right' (Loney, 1987). Its dogma accompanied the election of Margaret Thatcher's Conservative government in 1979. This movement stimulated a new creed and initiated a continuous set of deliberations that remain very alive and are unresolved to the present day. These consist of a trenchant critique containing political, economic and moral components about the overall ineffectiveness of the collective action that had given birth to and sustained the public services.

In ideological terms the welfare state and the British system of public services are seen by the New Right to be based on false assumptions. The idea that the state should attempt to provide equality of opportunity between individuals is regarded as an infeasible aspiration because it is held that individuals cannot be made better off or be improved morally simply by giving them a set of state-funded rights and entitlements. In essence, the New Right issued a rebuttal to conventional post-war thinking by openly declaring the notion of social justice to be an ethereal concept that is as impractical as it is unattainable.

The public services thus became branded paternalistic because they act on behalf of the individual in too many ways and had begun to assume responsibility for multifaceted aspects of people's personal lives. Such views argue that Britain's vast public service machinery constrains individual liberty through the lack of choice within the services that were available. State services came in a standardised form and alternative options to them were rarely available. Furthermore, it was argued that the extent of state involvement in the lives of individuals renders them passive, suppressed individual initiative and created a culture of dependency.

The New Right argue that, in realistic terms, there is no evidence that the welfare state has produced a more equitable and caring society; rather, that it has produced an underclass of individuals who are unable to act for themselves. This is evidenced as the welfare state's abject failure to deal with inequality and, furthermore, is believed to have created some of the very problems it set out to alleviate. Evidence proffered for this can be found in cases such as those people who are unemployed, who are caught in an earnings trap and are financially better off by living on state benefits than they would be in low-paid work.

The solution to all these criticisms is seen to lie in the return to a system that openly acknowledges that, first and foremost, relationships between people in a capitalist society are economic. What the New Right sees to be required is:

- The re-establishment of belief in the individual citizen as the focal point for political, economic and moral reasoning. This is necessary because the state cannot possibly assume collective responsibility for all of its individual citizens. Nor can the state identify what is the common good and then maintain the entitlement of individuals to a share of it. This gives way to claims that there is no such thing as society, only individuals.
- The reinstatement of the market principles of Adam Smith as a paramount requirement by allowing individuals to judge their own needs and wants. This concerns adherence to the laws of supply and demand and the primacy of free competition that must be unhindered by government interference.
- An emphasis on the individual as the sovereign consumer of goods and services. Consumers should be enabled to exercise free choice between commodities by expressing personal preferences through their personal spending decisions. It is believed that public services should be treated no differently from other consumer goods available in everyday life and that service users should be able to exercise the same sorts of judgements in acquiring, for example, their health care, as they employ when they purchase groceries.

THE ECONOMIC SYMBOLISM OF THE CONSERVATIVE YEARS, 1979–97

The 1979 Thatcher government initiated a train of events that continue to dominate economic policy and indeed much thinking about the way in which state welfare is provided both presently as well as in the future. The Labour government of the latter 1970s along with Keynesian economic policies began rapidly to lose their credibility with the electorate. There grew a broad agreement and a common feeling that far-reaching change was needed in the way the economy was managed and in the way that the country should be governed. Margaret Thatcher was elected in 1979 on a broad range of issues that aimed to restore public confidence in democratic government. The ideological starting point for the first administration was the strident resurrection of a set of traditional values that were reminiscent of the rhetoric of Victorian times. These emphasised the salience of such things as the significance of law and order and the institutional value of the family. All of this had a superficial attractiveness that appealed widely to the people because it appeared as an antidote to what many had previously perceived to be feeble government.

A new Conservative government brought with it a fresh economic policy that saw the introduction of the dogma of monetarist economic theory. As a consequence and as an adjunct to this, fresh thinking began to occur on the proper role of government in relation to public services as well as about the ways in which these should be paid for and delivered (Masich, 1983).

Monetarism was therefore adopted wholeheartedly and it remains the prominent mechanism for controlling the British economy; its introduction led to the rejection of the previous Keynesian approach to macroeconomic management. Monetarism argues that Keynesian economics had resulted in governments' interfering excessively with free-market exchange. The quest for full employment, high public expenditure and overall economic growth that had succeeded during the previous 30 years was seen to be failing substantially. Keynesian methods of managing the economy had produced high taxation but not the full employment or the economic growth needed to pay for ever-expanding public services. Monetarists argued that the approach had created high price inflation that was destroying the prosperity the people had come to expect. This was blamed for eroding the value of their personal savings and for suppressing the working capital of businesses.

Monetarism, or the quantity theory of money holds that:

- The key to economic growth and improved prosperity and better living standards relies on the control of inflation.
- This requires the Bank of England to strictly control the supply of money in circulation so that it does not exceed the expected growth in output. This requires careful economic forecasting so that the country lives effectively within its means.
- Monetarism contains the in-built supposition that management of the economy should not artificially maintain full employment and that

only economically sustainable jobs should exist. This is at variance with the former job-creation strategy that accompanied Keynesian economic thinking.

- Unemployment is therefore intended to find its own level. This belief from the early 1980s to the mid-1990s produced distress, and unemployment was believed necessary in the medium term to restore normal trading relationships with the rest of the world. These relationships were to eventually support the fuller employment that was indeed enjoyed at the end of the 1990s and at the commencement of the 21st century.

The political attractiveness of monetarism concerns its seeming simplicity (Johnson, 1991). When the Conservative government first introduced it in 1979 it starkly confronted those previously combative trade unions by presenting an option whereby they either accepted the level of wages that were on offer or faced the prospect of unemployment. Monetarism also provides a response to the accusations of state paternalism that are advanced by the New Right. It achieves this because it reduces overall political interference in the economy that requires only a light touch from the government of the day. The doctrine also finds wide acceptance with financial institutions because of the power it gives to them within the overall economy.

THE CONSERVATIVE YEARS AND THE MANAGEMENT OF THE PUBLIC SERVICES

The years between 1979 and 1997 saw continuous Conservative government that was steered politically by the ideology of the New Right and economically by monetarist economic theory. This represented an era marked initially by the reform of the previously unaccountable trade unions through legislation that limited their powers to disrupt British industry. The early part of the period was characterised by growing unemployment that began to weaken the formerly confrontational trade unions. A principal objective of the Thatcher administrations during the 1980s was to privatise government-owned industries. This was portrayed as the reduction of a burden on the taxpayer, a decrease in government interference in the way the country was run and a reduction of government intrusion into the lives of individuals, by enabling them to contract freely with private operators rather than being passive recipients of state services. The privatisation of large government-owned industries was accompanied by the flotation of shares in the newly privatised companies that also gave the people a notional new stake in the nation through the opportunity to become shareholders.

The 1979 Conservative government displayed a deep scepticism about state ownership in general and the welfare state in particular. It saw its task as one of reducing government intrusion in the economy wherever possible with the promotion of an enterprise culture where private ownership could flourish. While it was possible to attract capital from banks to privatise the more lucrative-looking state-controlled industries such as British Airways, the gas and telephone industries, some institutions of the welfare state were by no means as attractive to the owners of private capital.

CONSERVATIVE GOVERNMENTS AND THE NHS

The NHS is a prime example of a monolithic organisation that remained relatively unappealing to private capital and private investment. It is the largest employer in Europe with 1.3 million employees, one of the biggest employers in the world (Morris, 2003). Its building stock is very varied in its quality and some dates from the 19th century. The performance of its key functions, though consistently high, are very vulnerable to criticism in part because the NHS is so highly politicised. Although the post-war governments of both major persuasions have behaved in similar ways towards the NHS, each finds it possible to construct highly negative political capital about it when in opposition. These factors rendered only selective parts of it attractive to prospective private investors or buyers.

It can be seen that the NHS and most welfare state institutions therefore were not candidates for privatisation because their business is unpredictable and their environment is uncertain, and indeed risky, when judged by most common commercial criteria that concern profit and loss. Yet the NHS is a major cause of public spending. So its performance was highly significant to Conservative governments that had been elected on pledges to lower personal taxation and to lower public spending on services it saw to be inefficient. Solutions had to be sought. Although privatisation would have been the method of choice, compromises had to be sought during the Conservative years. Three major strategies were employed:

- a wholesale commitment to private provision;
- the use of contracting-out and of creeping privatisation strategies;
- the creation of quasi-markets or internal markets.

PRIVATISATION
The Conservative administrations between 1979 and 1997 were committed to the extension of private provision of public services wherever this

seemed economically possible and politically feasible. Notable examples include the subsidised sale of council housing. The pretext was that this would increase the number of owner-occupiers, who would take better care of their properties once they owned them that in turn would improve the housing stock and create the moral bonus of a property-owning democracy at the same time.

Private medical provision was also encouraged. Previous restrictions that required public consultation before a private hospital could be built were abolished and this saw a growth in private hospital provision. The key to private health care is private medical insurance and this saw a steady increase in subscribers that was most dramatic in the late 1970s and 1980s and achieved stability in the 1990s (ONS, 2002). A low of 2.1 million who were insured in 1971 grew to 6.9 million in 2000. This rise was entirely due to company-paid business because the number of individual private medical insurance subscribers fell between 1999 and 2000. This occurred because the Conservative Party gave tax allowances to retired people who had a health insurance policy in their former employment as an encouragement not to let their policy lapse once they ceased to work. New Labour, however, removed this when it was elected in 1997, causing many policies to lapse.

Hospital land sales and the sale of other unused assets also commenced to generate new forms of income from private sources. These income-generation projects ranged from the sale of redundant mental hospitals and other surplus land to the introduction of car parking fees at hospitals and the leasing of retail outlets in the foyers of NHS hospitals.

CONTRACTING-OUT AND CREEPING PRIVATISATION

Conservative governments also introduced the creeping privatisation by picking off those parts of the public services that were amenable to private competition. This was in harmony with the Tory view that the state might have an enduring responsibility to foot the bill for providing a particular service. That said, it need not necessarily remain a monopoly provider of it if a private organisation was able to compete against a traditional state-managed provider to deliver a superior product. Hotel services in hospitals were an early example of this principle where competitive tendering was introduced between in-house teams of cleaners, caterers and porters and outside private providers.

The privatisation of the long-term care of elderly people is a further example of how government relinquished its responsibility for providing intermediate and long-stay services but was willing to largely pay for the private sector to provide them. Historically, the state had a range of provision for the long-term care of elderly people. This consisted of NHS geriatric hospital and psycho-geriatric hospital provision and elderly care homes run by local authorities. The 1980s saw a move to privatise this type of care in old age as far as and wherever possible. Dedicated hospital beds were reduced and geriatric hospitals and the psycho-geriatric facilities were closed. Patients were transferred to rest homes and the state pension and benefit regulations were amended to make elderly people's benefit entitlements available to pay for their residential home and nursing home care. Means testing was introduced and those elderly people with assets began to have to use their savings and, in some cases, sell their homes to fund care that had been provided previously by the state. Similarly, local authority homes were sold off or closed and their residents transferred to the private residential home sector. A new definition of care known as 'social care' appeared for which it could be argued was a euphemism for those aspects of care for which individuals with means would be charged for what, formerly, were free public services.

QUASI- OR INTERNAL MARKETS

The White Paper *Working for Patients* paved the way for the NHS and Community Care Act 1990 and initiated the idea of the internal market in health and social care, and this impacted on the NHS and on local authorities (DOH, 1989). The key feature of this arrangement is the purchaser/provider split. Central to this means of dealing is the idea of contracting. The elements of the contract are that:

- a provider agrees to deliver for the purchaser a particular volume of service;
- at a particular price and quality;
- by a particular time.

Under this system local authorities became purchasers of social care and health authorities became purchasers of hospital care and treatment. Local authorities were compelled to purchase care from providers who were either profit-making private care organisations such as residential homes, or from the increasing number of non-profit-making charitable organisations. These latter organisations proliferated to plug gaps in public provision for groups like the former residents of long-stay mental and learning disability hospitals.

Health authorities had originally managed their local hospitals as well as purchasing the care for them. The internal market created a new set of relationships. Health authorities became purchasers and hospitals became providers and were given a new semi-autonomous status by being designated as NHS trusts. In reality, despite some freedoms such as the limited right to raise private capital, they remained subject to stringent government controls.

This method of internal market organisation was meant to mimic the operation of free commercial markets and to do so within services that were to remain largely state financed. Organisations like the NHS and local authorities had always understood what their total annual cost was. What was new about the internal market was the requirement to determine the detailed price of individual elements of service: for example, the price of an individual surgical operation. Having detailed pricing information was an essential prerequisite to the development of the quasi-trading relationship and to the introduction of the notion of competition into the public services. It is the price mechanism that powers those free commercial markets that the public services were intended to emulate; this can be understood at its basic level as follows:

- the spontaneous demand for a commodity or a service will produce a price rise;
- a price rise will usually give providers of a service an incentive to increase their profits so this stimulates extra production;
- extra production results in the relief of scarcity;

To transfer this last analogy to the NHS it can be seen that:

- a spontaneous rise in the number of patients needing hip replacement operations should stimulate an NHS trust to be able to ask a higher price because of the demand;
- orthopaedic teams in the NHS trust should therefore have an incentive to operate on more patients to increase their income and hence their profit;
- the increased surgical activity should mean that the waiting list for hip replacement should be reduced thus reducing the scarcity of care for the procedure.

This over-simplistic explanation tells little about the true complexities of advanced capitalist economies. Yet free-market thinking contends that a system of exchange on the basis of an agreed price maintains its own equilibrium and allocates resources efficiently. At one level, therefore, the rationale for internal markets in health care stemmed from the ideology that central government-driven decisions are inferior to private individual decisions in delivering public services. The argument goes that markets behave spontaneously and are capable of reacting more rapidly to changing need within public service organisations than the traditional funding methods used by local authorities or the NHS. It was envisaged that a system of competition would be created between providers that would weed out inefficiency and would produce smooth change within organisations. Strong providers would survive and prosper while weaker providers would wither and go out of business.

THE EXPERIENCE OF THE INTERNAL MARKET IN HEALTH CARE, 1990–97

The idea of an internal market in health care originated in the work of an American health economist Alain Enthoven (Enthoven, 1985). This was translated by the Conservative governments of the 1990s into a working policy and a set of quasi-trading practices designed to improve the delivery of health services through a purchaser/provider split. Another phenomenon, that was not Enthoven's creation, was also introduced that was known as GP (general practitioner) fundholding, whereby some GPs were able to purchase care directly from NHS trusts. The core principle in this arrangement was that money would follow the patient, thus giving providers a new incentive to treat more patients. Enthoven subsequently produced an analysis of the effects of these internal market reforms in the NHS (Enthoven, 1999).

   The internal market probably did produce more productivity and introduced a culture of more business-like cost-consciousness into the NHS but its success was limited by a number of crucial issues. Competition, which was intended to be economically more efficient, produce higher quality services and send the weakest providers to the wall, did not flourish, because the infrastructure for these things to occur did not exist. Other handicapping factors were as follows:

* To produce competition required a large investment in information technology, contract managers and accountants. This generated higher administrative costs that were compounded by a convoluted, bureaucratic and expensive system of invoicing that impacted negatively on the financial benefits of improved productivity.
* The market information and details of pricing needed to produce genuine trading relationships was poor, resulting in weak market forces.
* Pricing information lacked transparency so that competing providers did not have access to the prices of their rivals.
* Health authority purchasers or GPs acted as a proxy for the patients. Patients therefore did not have the information to make rational economic decisions about their care so that the true notion of consumer choice failed to develop.

- Purchasers continued to buy from their local supplier as they always had done and there was little evidence of them shopping around for the best buy.
- For some NHS trusts in geographically remote parts there was no one with whom to compete. Something resembling a competitive market was possible in large cities that had more than one provider but the Conservative government managed competition because it was afraid of the political controversy that might result if particular services that were cherished locally had to be reduced or closed.
- NHS trusts had such low reserves of working capital that it would have been easy for a large GP fundholder to destabilise the market simply by moving business from a local hospital to a provider elsewhere. This was a further reason for government to manage the internal market.
- Patients followed the contract, rather than money following the patient, and contracts were rarely removed from weak provider trusts so that even seriously failing providers were allowed to stay in business.
- There was the potential for patients of GP fundholders to fare better than those of non-fundholder patients, creating inequities in the access to services.

The Conservative years created an impression that the welfare state was being dismantled. Certainly, attitudes to it changed and so the superiority of totally publicly funded health and social care services was challenged both ideologically and practically. A bigger private element in welfare provision had appeared. Consumerism became the watchword and although government interference in the operational management of services had been strengthened, there was little evidence that individual citizens were genuinely empowered. Attitudes within public service institutions were nevertheless transformed through the values and practices derived from private business that were adopted in the quest for greater efficiency. But rather than being abandoned, the welfare state remained largely intact and changed its shape rather than its fundamental purpose.

NEW LABOUR AND THE CONTINUING DEBATE ABOUT PUBLIC SERVICES IN BRITAIN FROM 1997 INTO THE 21ST CENTURY

New Labour came to power in May 1997 within a public mood resembling that which welcomed the first Thatcher government in 1979. The electorate was reasonably unequivocal that it was time for a change, and the first administration of Tony Blair was given a strong mandate at the ballot box and his second government was returned to power for a second term in June 2001 with an even greater majority. The size of their electoral lead was such that it potentially gave the second New Labour government the power to create unbridled change. In the course of both terms of office New Labour abandoned, incrementally, many of the party's time-honoured socialist principles concerning collectivist state provision and committed itself to what historically had been the Conservative Party's philosophy. Most notably it stuck to the monetarist doctrine of the Tories and adhered faithfully to its predecessor's policy not to increase personal taxation and to keep spending on public services under control. In theory, New Labour held on to the belief that services such as the NHS should be regarded as a public good to which all in employment are willing to sub-scribe. At the same time, however, New Labour did not hesitate to main-tain Tory market principles and, indeed, in some instances (such as the Private Finance Initiative) it expanded the use of them. This was in direct contradiction to the Party's traditional stance on public services and it has been contended that New Labour became progressively Thatcherite (Warden, 1998).

New Labour's 1997 manifesto contained strong claims that it would abandon quasi-markets in health care. In 1997 it immediately set about doing this in principle, but in reality it left a great many previously created Conservative structures and procedures relatively untouched. In effect it set about coining New Labour terminology for what had been the previous Conservative government's procedures and practices. New Labour claimed to have discarded the internal market in health care. Yet it retained the purchaser/provider split and while allegedly having forsaken contracting, which is the central feature of the quasi-trading process, it actually renamed the deal struck between the purchaser and the provider to be a 'service-level agreement'. By 2003, during its second term, New Labour had not only restored the Conservative internal market model of health care through the creation of fundholding primary care trusts (PCTs) but it had gone far beyond Tory achievements with plans to enable hospitals to opt out of state control.

From an early juncture, New Labour had to acknowledge covertly that the ideology of the welfare state and its system of public services that had been put in place following World War II was becoming difficult to sustain because the demands made upon them were infinite. At the same time it had to appease its traditionalists from the 'Old Labour' tradition on its left wing. There was nevertheless a general acceptance of the typical Conservative Party view that the system of public provision produces a dependency culture. New Labour therefore envisaged that solutions to the deficiencies in public services would be found in the following:

- Remedying social and economic failure that created a dependency culture by reducing unemployment.
- Improving the targeting of services and dealing more strictly with fraud through better surveillance and the enforcement of the rules of entitlement to state services.
- Improved means testing.
- Encouraging greater self-reliance and promoting self-sufficiency.
- Reconciling policies from both the right and the left that were previously seen to be antagonistic through the adoption of its doctrine known as the 'Third Way'. The doctrine of the Third Way holds that it is possible to embrace long-established Labour thinking about social justice whilst simultaneously employing free-market principles to secure its political ends (Blair, 1998).

What emerged was a consensus view from the major parties that these services cannot be sustained in perpetuity in their current form. The public services in Britain have a high political profile and governments of all persuasions have responded typically to service shortages by allocating money to them generously as a means to a quick political resolution. The issue for New Labour, therefore, is simply not one of investment in services but concerns the ways in which modernisation is to be achieved and a long-term strategy fashioned. The key questions to achieve these things concern:

- What is the optimum means of paying for health services in the longer term?
- Who will be the most appropriate providers?

The New Labour government retained its commitment to services that are funded predominantly from the public purse (HM Treasury, 2002a). But it increasingly moved towards the views of the strongest critics of state-funded services in its commitment to notions of choice, competition and privatisation. The views of these critics were typified by the work of the Adam Smith Institute (ASI) whose founding principles can be seen to coincide in some respects with New Labour's public service policies (Browne and Young, 2002). So even if the funding base for health care does not change, the mechanisms of delivery are patently intended to do so.

   The ASI is Britain's leading proponent of market economic policies and has played a key role in the analysis and development of public policies through the publication of many influential policy reports. The organisation has been part of a worldwide movement towards free markets and free trade. The ASI's objective is for the public to have options and for there to be open competition between providers. This is the essence of a free market that is intended to empower ordinary people by giving them the chance to help frame their future by their direct involvement and the expression of choices. It is believed that through consumer choice public services will be redesigned in ways that inject innovation and customer responsiveness into their delivery. The ASI begins from the somewhat extreme position that in its current form the welfare state is pathological (Marsland, 1994). It believes that the welfare state and the public services it provides have:

- become archaic because these were designed for economic circumstances when Britain was an industrial nation that differ from those that prevail in the 21st century;
- diverted money away from economic growth in ways that impairs investment in the economy;
- reduced personal freedom and choice by causing excessive, compulsory personal taxation over which individuals have absolutely no control either over the amount by which they are taxed or over how their contribution is used by government;
- failed to eliminate poverty;
- suppressed personal initiative, stifled independence and prevented individuals acting for themselves;
- created an underclass from which there is no chance of escape;
- resulted in bureaucratic institutional structures that are inefficient and offer mediocre services;
- resulted in state paternalism.

These sentiments support a safety net of services for a small minority but contend that many public services should be largely replaced by private provision in which the prosperous majority would be encouraged to insure for sickness, education and for pensions. It can be seen from such propositions that consumer choice as well as the adequate financing of services is crucial to their modernisation and it becomes arguable that the current state-financed services spend money inappropriately and fail to deliver what the population actually wants (Butler and Pirie, 2001).

So clearly, as a starting point, New Labour sought to ensure services that are available through general taxation but its stance was that it does not need to control every aspect of their delivery. It took the view therefore that public services need to be restructured to accommodate individual preference and that only when alternatives are available so that individuals can express their likes and dislikes will the publicly funded services improve in terms of their efficiency and quality.

Different sources of provision are thus seen to be required as alternatives to those publicly funded services to add variety and give choice to the consumer. This means that the supply of services could come legitimately from private profit-making organisations, charitable organisations and not-for-profit organisations as well as from existing public providers. In keeping with its Conservative Party predecessors, New Labour believed that competition is the principal feature of such arrangements because by making service users into consumers, they will exert their own vested interests. This will sequentially drive up quality standards. Furthermore, genuine competition stimulates innovation and newer providers have incentives to enter the market with novel responses to old challenges and with a commitment to achieve the highest standards. In the last resort, those parts of the conventional public services adjudged to be inefficient or failing their clientele such as under-performing hospital trusts would be closed or their business put out to competitive tender.

THE NEW LABOUR APPROACH TO PUBLIC SERVICE PROVISION

New Labour occupied an interesting piece of political ground. Until the mid-1990s Old Labour was passionately committed to social justice and the collectivist provision of public services. It vigorously opposed the strategies of Thatcherism that saw an increased role for individual wealth creation and a withdrawal of government from the provision of state services. New Labour retained a notional commitment to social justice but has sufficed to redefine it through the creation of its 'Third Way' (Giddens, 1998). This innovation provides an amalgam of the two earlier doctrines of the Old Left and the New Right. Through the Third Way, New Labour sought to reconcile those two former polarities by embracing notions of the left such as the need for equality, equity and redistribution yet it accepted, concurrently, right-wing mechanisms for achieving these through private market mechanisms (Blair, 1998). Old Labour had been an outright champion of publicly provided services and rejected everything within Tory thinking that advocated the dismantling of the welfare state. By contrast, while supporting public provision out of necessity, New Labour was happy to see the private delivery of services in ways that are perfectly acceptable to the Conservative Party. The 'Third Way' thus provided a doctrine to sustain a new model of service provision that contained a mixed, public and private economy. Three interrelated and overlapping factors constitute its conceptual basis, namely:

- creating consumer involvement and choice;
- stimulating provider rivalry and competition;
- setting standards of excellence.

The Third Way advocates a series of the free-market assumptions about the absence of competition between the existing and potentially new providers of public services. When government agencies purchase public services they usually do so from the top down, beginning with decisions in the spending departments of the government. This secures services that are provided at the same or a similar level of quality for all users who have few or usually no alternatives. The NHS epitomises this position. A patient needing an expert opinion visits a GP who refers the patient to the local consultant and usually no choice is available to the patient. The NHS user gets what is on offer. This state of affairs has been referred to as 'producer capture' because production is dominated by government, the purchaser of the product or, in this instance, the patient forfeits the ability to shop around for a better buy (Pirie and Worcester, 2001). This inevitably means that the interests of central government policy transcend those of service users. Unlike failing private providers, failing providers of public services such as NHS hospitals do not go into liquidation. In consequence, there is really no economic incentive for them to provide anything other than the basic essentials within their standard service (Butler and Pirie, 2001).

CREATING CONSUMER CHOICE

New Labour has thus re-emphasised the Conservative idea of creating scope for user selection within state provision. To date, new notions of consumerism within public services have improved the providers' understandings of user expectations, yet individuals still have no real means at their disposal for changing the essentials of the services they will receive. New Labour thinking therefore argues that users must become consumers. As consumers, choices are made between various producers, and the real consumer strives to maximise the best possible value for money. Consumer sovereignty is the dogma underpinning each transaction whereby opinions and choices of the individual become the paramount concerns of providers. Accordingly, New Labour envisaged a similar model being available within public services whereby users should have options as to where to locate their business. Consumer choice, where funding follows the consumer, gives new incentives to providers, be they public or private, to respond to the needs and wants of those they serve and to appeal to as many of them as possible in order to boost their returns.

STIMULATING PROVIDER RIVALRY AND COMPETITION

New Labour was reluctant to use the term 'competition' to identify commercial rivalry between providers because of its overtly Thatcherite connotations and so it tended to describe it euphemistically as 'contestability'

(DOH, 2003a). In keeping with this tendency to introduce its own lexicon it preferred to refer to 'public–private partnerships' to the more forthright term 'privatisation'.

The competitive element therefore became evident within the spirit if not the letter of New Labour public services policy that emphasised the promotion of a new commercial-style culture (DOH, 2002a). Terminology aside, it is a generally accepted maxim that within free-market trading arrangements businesses exist primarily to make money and to increase the yield of their shareholders. But to do so they must not only respond to the wishes of their clients but must also anticipate their prospective needs in order to provide new, improved products. Commercial organisations, unlike state-provided public services, fend off competitors to secure a market share in order to stay alive in the market place. It is this affinity with the client in the overall cause to achieve greater economic success that New Labour sought to mimic in the delivery of social goods and services. While this cannot possibly provide a true replication of the economic decisions an individual takes when purchasing in the typical market place, it nevertheless provides a template for market-oriented behaviour to which New Labour wished its public services to aspire.

SETTING STANDARDS OF EXCELLENCE

Government acts as an understudy for the taxpayer in providing public services. This means that the taxpayer loses all control over the destiny of a resource that has been earned personally. The government monopolises the distribution of most public services and the place of providers has been secure because they have not had to compete. The internal market in health care in the 1990s envisaged some competition. But poor pricing information and over-regulation by government meant that its effects were limited. This control of provision has meant that it is highly difficult for the benefactor of those services, namely the taxpayer, to evaluate their functioning and their overall value to society at large.

New Labour therefore aimed to reduce dependency and to empower consumers of services through better information. It began this by subtly employing policies that have their origins in decidedly free-market sources of opinion (DOH, 2002a; Butler and Pirie, 2001; Pirie and Worcester, 2001).

Labour's embrace of the thinking that is in tandem with Thatcherism has been demonstrated as follows, through:

- a substantial extension of the private finance initiative (PFI) to build new hospitals and also to upgrade GP premises through local improvement finance trusts (LIFT);

- the use of under-occupancy of private hospital beds to treat NHS patients requiring paying for elective surgery under its concordat with the private sector (DOH, 2002a, 2002b);
- the introduction of NHS-purchased intermediate care to relieve delayed discharges that were provided for elderly people in the privately run nursing home and rest home sector;
- the increased empowerment of frontline staff and a commitment to let them make the vast majority of spending decisions in the NHS through the creation of PCTs (DOH, 2002a);
- the creation of NHS foundation trust hospitals that are independent not-for-profit organisations that are outside the control of the Department of Health (DOH, 2002c);
- the recruitment of private companies from overseas to increase NHS capacity in the provision of diagnostic and elective surgical services (DOH, 2002b).

The next predictable steps were that private sector providers will be invited to take over failing NHS services such as the first failing NHS foundation hospital trust (Butler and Pirie, 2001; Wilkinson, 2003).

TOWARDS THE FUTURE

It can be seen that the dilemmas in modernising public service provision come back to the recurrent debate that is two-fold. Firstly, how will be services be funded and, secondly, how and by whom will they be delivered?

FUNDING THE PUBLIC SERVICES

In the longer term there is a serious debate about the balance between collective responsibility and individual responsibility in providing personal services to meet human needs. This discussion concerns the balance between those things it is reasonable to expect the state to provide and those that the individual might justly be expected to provide from private economic means.

There are some aspects of the welfare state such as unemployment benefit where there is probably little scope for market solutions. But in other areas such as medical insurance and private health care there is the possibility for a more substantial private–public mix of funding sources. There are other models available that combine public and private, payments and insurance in France and Germany that are worthy of further study. This means that if people want different levels of service, for instance, it is possible to top up a basic state entitlement by using personal savings. Clearly there need to be safety measures in place for the low paid, the poor and those who are uninsurable. Most countries in Europe have shown such systems can work well and with fairness. What is predictable is that a great many services that were funded by the state at the end of the 20th century will probably be beyond its financial means by 2020, given the changing demographic structure and the diminishing number of taxpayers who will be in employment to support a growing elderly population through payment of their taxes.

In the shorter term, governments seem set to have the bulk of public services funded from the public purse (HM Treasury, 2002a; Duncan Smith, 2003). The debate therefore shifts to one about who should deliver them. The New Labour manifesto of 2001 made a clear commitment to reform and rebuild Britain's public services (Labour Party, 2001). The question is one of means rather than ends and this immediately opens up a long-standing argument about the greater use by government of both private financing and the private delivery of public services.

A MIXED ECONOMY IN PUBLIC SERVICE DELIVERY

A balance therefore is being struck between the state and the non-state sectors (Butler and Yarrow, 2001). Little is known about the potential relative contribution of public sector and private sector provision and how these might become synergistic. It is therefore not so much a matter of either predominantly public solutions or predominantly private ones, rather one of deciding what either provides most appropriately and what is best provided in partnership.

What is predictable is that any mention of private involvement in the provision of public services is likely to be interpreted by some as a move to dismantle the welfare state. This assumes that increased private involvement will occur only in the interests of private providers and will necessarily work to the detriment of public provision (Harrison, 2001). What has not been properly estimated is the scope that is offered by the creation of a mixed economy in public services. A mixed economy offers the state the opportunity to convert the users of services into consumers. What seems certain is that the extent of private involvement in provision is merely in embryonic form and seems certain to grow with the potential that the state could, eventually, become merely the residual regulator of the volume and quality of services.

CONCLUSION

This chapter has addressed some of the ideological, political and economic precursors for today's NHS. It can be seen that the consensus on whether public services should be collectively funded and provided has been breaking up gradually for almost three decades. The main debates have been circular in nature with New Labour gradually shedding its old socialist dogma and taking a stance closely resembling that characterising the Conservative governments of the 1990s.

The vast majority of the British public has grown up to have pride in and to wholeheartedly support the institutions of the welfare state and the ethical precepts that underpin it. Arguments that these institutions can be easily reformed are difficult to sustain. Those who support this point of view generally claim it is just a question of money, but that is just the start.

The public service institutions in Britain of which the NHS is the archetype are the last of the central command organisations in existence. In recent times they have been managed by a central government that dictates the minutiae of their everyday activities. This has occurred through a myriad of complicated targets and initiatives that confound even those who are charged to implement them. It can be seen how monolithic institutions such as the NHS might be modernised is an intricate and politically explosive matter. What is certain is that modernisation is needed and governments will continue to introduce untried reforms in the interest of change of which improvement will be a much-valued outcome.

The following chapter will address the modernisation agenda for the NHS that emanates from the time of the 1997 New Labour government.

TWO

THE MODERNISATION AGENDA OF THE NHS

This chapter will build on the factors identified in Chapter 1. In particular it will address the prolific modernisation plans that were commenced following the election of New Labour in 1997. This state of change seems likely to continue relentlessly for the foreseeable future irrespective of which government is in office because all the major parties are committed to their own version of NHS reform.

A UNIQUE SET OF INTENTIONS

The NHS brought order out of chaos. It was conceived in the early 1940s and introduced in 1948 because the British health care system prior to World War II was in a state of disarray. Health care had been uncoordinated. It was delivered inefficiently, its supply was inequitable geographically and the entire system was close to financial collapse. At the outbreak of war in 1939 over half the population, mainly women and children, were without health insurance cover. In practice, wealthier people paid for their care and treatment and entered the front door of the consulting room by appointment. The lower social classes were admitted to the surgery door and obliged to wait their turn (Whitehead, 1994). A fact of life for the less privileged, therefore, was that they lived in fear of illness not least of all because they dreaded how they might pay doctors' bills.

In 1952, during the early life of the service, 50 per cent of the population still lived in areas that had an inadequate number of doctors to reasonably meet their needs. This remains a lesser though enduring problem in inner cities where general practice is not immediately appealing to doctors despite the financial incentives that are offered to attract them there.

The minister of health at the inception of the NHS was Aneurin Bevan, who built and articulated the equity principles on which the NHS was to be constructed (Foot, 1999). These were meant to address the wide variation in both the availability and the quality of these early services. The principles of equity on which the NHS was founded remain and it is these values that render it unique internationally. They comprise:

- universal access;
- services that are free at the point of delivery;
- an inclusive range of services for all health needs from the cradle to the grave;
- selection on the basis of clinical need that does not depend on the ability to pay;
- the provision of equality of geographical access, parity of standards and a spread of supra-regional specialities that is comprehensive and cost effective;
- dependence on revenue that is raised from general taxation that can be collected from those in work and redistributed to those with service needs with administrative and economic efficiency;
- strict central control of major capital developments to ensure that facilities are developed where they produce the best return for their financial outlay;
- a strong primary care system that produces fewer hospital admissions than in many other similar countries;
- a strong democratic commitment to the NHS by the British people (Enthoven, 1991; Whitehead, 1994).

Governments of all persuasions have signed up to and continue to adhere to these bold aspirations. Yet some critics of the NHS would contend that, despite its beneficent intentions, the aims and beliefs on which it was founded have become outmoded. Opponents suppose that the levels of access, comprehensiveness and fairness that are espoused for the service have become entirely unachievable. According to this point of view, the pursuit of equity through such mechanisms as universal access to health care is believed to make individuals dependent on the state to the extent that they even eschew responsibility for their own health (Marsland, 1994).

Equity in health care concerns the fair or just distribution of services to those who need them and this provides an overwhelming ethos and a source of motivation to those professionals on whose goodwill the NHS relies in order to function efficiently. Yet the concept of equity has tended to be associated with equality, which is not quite the same thing. Equality is the equal distribution of shares so that each individual receives the same arithmetical amount of a particular commodity (Pariera, 1989). The search for equality in the provision of health care has been regarded by governments to be inappropriate because people are not born with equal health status, their lifestyles differ and the health needs of individuals change over time. So, despite these highly honourable policy intentions, the concept of equity does assume that a reasonable degree of inequality is unavoidable. But in accepting this, governments seek ways to minimise it and improve the justness in the ways services are distributed. It is when services are seen to be distributed unfairly, however, that the highly politicised nature of the NHS is at its most apparent.

A HIGHLY POLITICISED SERVICE

The political problems caused to governments by the NHS are inevitable. The NHS holds a precious place in the imagination of the British people and it serves to unite them. It has been claimed that its standing is comparable even to that of a religion and that this suppresses the debate about it that is really required (Neuberger, 1999). It can be seen, therefore, that the overall condition of the NHS and the government's standing with the public are closely intertwined (Davies, 2003). It is politicians themselves who suggest that more health services mean better health, and this reinforces the high political profile of health care. It means usually that the NHS is among the top three issues at any general election with only war and unemployment guaranteed to be ahead of it in terms of its electoral importance. The people thus believe that better services produce better health outcomes and this shapes their expectations and leads them to assume that medicine can always do something extraordinary. These idealistic perceptions sometimes hinder the recognition that, although organised medicine is clearly important, its real achievements can be elevated to a point of exaggeration. What is evident is that the service is scourged by delay and by variable outcomes for patients (Stationery Office, 2001a).

This basic political problem is intensified by the double-edged nature of the demands made for services that will always exceed their supply. Access is easy because the NHS is free at the point of delivery and there are few disincentives for those who seek to use it. In addition, the comprehensiveness of what is on offer means that demand also arises from suppliers and an aggressive pharmaceutical industry, and even from innovative staff who wish to introduce new techniques. Furthermore, new clinical advances are usually more expensive than those they replace. Government also fuels the politicisation through a commitment to provide high quality standards of care and treatment that are available nation-wide.

So after over half a century since the birth of the NHS, it can still be confirmed that three of the policy precepts on which the service was founded (namely, free access to services, their comprehensive range and their high quality) are alive and well and are still being pursued with vigour (DOH, 2002d). Yet these elemental policies can be seen to be mutually antagonistic. For instance, to secure the best clinical outcome for some patients post-operatively, it might be necessary to set a length of in-patient stay that will sacrifice access to others who are waiting for a bed to become available. Conversely, sending the patient home early would free the bed for additional use but might be judged to lessen the quality of care to the patient. By providing a fully comprehensive service that is freely available to all means that the cheaper, less effective, treatment options might have to be selected on occasions that will also threaten the quality of service. The pursuit of the highest quality service that is universal and is also free will similarly pose threats to the breadth of services that are available threatening comprehensiveness. This means that some services such as *in vitro* fertilisation are not freely available to those who wish for it and have, until recently, had to be purchased privately.

The NHS is thus the victim of its own success, and because it is highly politicised opposition politicians of any persuasion are always in a position to capitalise on its perceived deficiencies. Because we have exceeded our ability to afford all the care and treatment that is available it is not difficult to portray the NHS as an organisation that is in a state of chronic crisis, and politicians in opposition profit from this to their advantage (Dixon and Harrison, 1997).

NHS REORGANISATIONS

The NHS has been restructured regularly throughout its history. This is also the case in modern times where the specific intention is to make it more efficient and accountable. Two observations can be made on the issues of reform, restructuring and reorganisation. Firstly, the evidence suggests that there are few examples where the wholesale organisational change that has occurred contains ideas that are entirely new (Ham, 1999). This is indeed the case for what New Labour branded the 'New NHS' because it used renamed versions of the market-oriented policies of the previous Conservative government. Secondly, most reorganisations have shown that the NHS is remarkably impervious to either ideological or funding changes and it withstands these in ways that demonstrate very little evidence of measurable transformation. Rather the adjustments that do occur are at a level of presentation and rhetoric rather than of genuine substance (Klein, 1998).

Four distinct versions of structural change during the life of the NHS have been described (Powell, 2000). These are:·

- **Central command and control.** This approach relies on central planning and assumes that the government can judge the health needs of the nation through the aggregation of regional plans. Having collated the necessary information it then attempts to distribute resources with sufficient precision to meet the needs that have been defined. This was the preferred approach of the early NHS, and although devolved management responsibility has increased, command and control still exists as evidenced by the frequency with which successive secretaries of state have engaged themselves in the minutiae of local health affairs.
- **The restructured NHS of the 1980s.** The government of Margaret Thatcher spent the decade attempting to find new solutions to the original command and control model and to make it work better. This era sought greater efficiency as it removed surplus tiers of management to reduce bureaucracy. It introduced chief executives to hospitals with ultimate accountability for their performance. Techniques of industrial-style management were initiated and these were intended to speed up and improve the accuracy of decision making. Hotel and catering services were contracted out to private suppliers of catering, laundry, cleaning and portering services to secure more financial efficiency.
- **The NHS market of the 1990s.** The White Paper *Working for Patients* was the landmark publication that heralded the introduction of the internal market in health care (DOH, 1989). This was to bring in hitherto unprecedented change in the ways in which the NHS managed its transactions. Health authorities and GP fundholders became the *purchasers* of care and were split organisationally from NHS trust hospitals that became labelled as the *providers* of care and treatment. The intention of this policy was to increase economic efficiency through competition and, as can be seen from Chapter 1 (page 15), this failed to materialise successfully.
- **New Labour and the new NHS.** The 1997 New Labour government was committed to abandon the internal market. But after cosmetically removing some of its features in its first term, it proceeded in its second term after 2001 to pursue market principles in a disguised form with a zest that far surpassed that of the former Conservative government. It can be seen, however, that New Labour did set a range of highly ambitious targets and emphasised the notion of patient involvement and consumerism in a fashion that was unprecedented.

NEW LABOUR AND THE POLITICS OF NHS CHANGE

New Labour set out its intentions for the NHS by asserting that the service was the principal dividing line between itself and the Conservatives in its preparation for the 1997 general election (Harman, 1996). Its overall strategy was couched within the rubric of its canon known as the 'third way', and this gave direction to policies that were designed to develop, reinforce and modernise the NHS (Giddens, 1998).

New Labour's approach to reform became increasingly radical as its period in office progressed. It seemed in 1997 to be taking a minimalist approach to alter the service. Previous experience from the earlier 1990s provided confirmation that NHS reform is often approached with dogmatic aims that eventually become unworkable. What originates as a scheme to save money has a curious knack of costing substantially more than was envisaged originally. For instance, the cost of the administrative overhead at the creation of the internal market in 1991 by the Conservative government was 8.8 per cent of total expenditure (Harman, 1996). But the system brought with it increasing bureaucracy resulting from a complicated costly system of invoicing. Harman cited the case of the United Leeds Teaching Hospital Trust that had 300 separate contracts a year with its purchasing health authority, all to be monitored regularly and renewed annually. During this work the trust issued 12,500 invoices a year and it was estimated that, by 1996, this system wasted £1.5 billion per annum nationally and accounted for 11.9 per cent of the total NHS budget and had created 20,000 more managers and 50,000 fewer nurses (Harman, 1996).

Moreover, most reorganisations that are intended to make economies usually claim to reduce management costs, but what savings they do secure are often offset by the early retirement and redundancy packages that are necessary to dispose of staff who are surplus to requirements. It has been argued that, between 1993 and 2003, the NHS has experienced financial growth in real terms of 45 per cent but that this has been misdirected to support the proliferating bureaucracy that evolved to set and monitor the targets that had been set by New Labour (Slevin, 2003). This assertion was accompanied by the allegation that the service has almost as many managers as it does registered nurses. In comparison to the private hospital sector, the 'manager to registered nurse' ratio is four and a half times higher in the NHS (Slevin, 2003). In considering this assertion it seems only fair also to recognise that private hospitals are usually far less complex organisations to manage than NHS hospitals.

In initiating its NHS reforms New Labour's approach to demand differed from anything the service has experienced previously. The NHS has survived over time by employing a model for the formation of its health policies that has been described as technocratic paternalism (Klein, 1995). This has assumed that professionals, especially the medical profession, know best and that service users are in a state of relative ignorance that results in their expectations not being canvassed and certainly not being raised. The consequence of this is that there has been little pressure on the NHS to do things much differently than it has always done them. In its first term New Labour began tentatively with reference to meeting patient needs (DOH, 1997). But after its re-election in 2001 its stance had become palpably more consumer oriented. In examples such as access to treatment and patient choice, for instance, it seemed to know not only what the people need, which is a tall enough order in its own right, but it also began to advocate for them to express their preferences (DOH, 2003a). It is true that there is an increasingly discerning public that is not willing to tolerate the institutional deference some NHS professionals have expected of it and who are probably less tolerant of having to wait than their predecessors. Yet New Labour embarked on a programme that set modernisation targets for the NHS to meet and linked these to a new accountability to the public through a set of standards and performance indicators that differentiate stronger performing parts of the organisation from their weaker counterparts.

This suggests strong central direction through a doctrinaire political line from the secretary of state for health, through the NHS Executive to the chairs of strategic health authorities and then to chairs of primary care and NHS trusts. This has meant that the centre formulated policy. Its Executive vetted local plans and had strategic health authorities to monitor their implementation. All of this has assumed an expectation that local management and local clinicians would gladly endorse and enthusiastically follow government edicts. The successful delivery of services at the local level thus became judged by short-term, bottom-line targets that were determined by political imperatives. A performance management system operated, designed to identify failings in local trusts so that sanctions could be taken against those that did not succeed. This represented a policy that failed to accept that some organisations have to be at the bottom of the league table. Superficially, therefore, government seemed to be in control. But this may not have been the most suitable means to achieve the intended end. Indeed there has been a literature extending back over 30 years that argues that rigorous performance management through strict arithmetical target setting and the use of performance-related pay, with penalties being taken against those who fail, is an inefficient means of initiating change (Deming, 1968). An alternative approach is to nurture those in prominent management positions and to defend them fully when times are difficult. However, this was in direct contrast to the New Labour approach that set out to name and shame those adjudged to be performing least well.

In the final analysis it might be supposed that the failure to come up to particular standards was a responsibility of local management, and that certainly became the case. Government blamed local managers when everything did not go to plan. But that did not necessarily absolve government from the accusation that its overall plans might have been over-ambitious in the first place, or that some services will just lack the capacity to meet the intended target. So despite New Labour's heavy financial investment in meeting its overabundance of NHS targets, it did nevertheless leave itself a hostage to political fortune if it was seen to fail to deliver substantially on all of those things it promised so faithfully.

THE NHS PLAN: THE BLUEPRINT FOR THE FUTURE

The *NHS Plan* of July 2000 was the landmark starting point for New Labour's massive 10-year reform of the NHS (DOH, 2000a, 2000b, 2000c). It in turn gave way to a welter of subsequent policy documents that concerned the implementation of the *Plan* (www.doh.gov.uk). The policy embodied an unmatched vision and was accompanied by an unsurpassed increase in funding. But as the strategy unfolded and the *Plan* began to be put into operation the difficulties in achieving tangible improvement in the performance of the NHS became apparent. This raised questions about how effective organisational change on this scale in a public service of the sheer size of the NHS, could be achieved realistically.

The NHS is a convoluted organisation comprising many different groups with varied vested interests. In this regard it is unlike most other large commercial organisations, although over the last 20 years there has been a tendency for governments to assume it is just another business. It differs from commercial companies in major respects. Its primary motive is service to people rather than profit. Its beneficiaries are its patients rather than its shareholders and it is resourced largely from general taxation so that in part it is accountable to the electorate. In a production-line industry the end product is clear to see as a number of specific products whereas the NHS has far less tangible outputs. Much of what it does is less easy to define in concrete terms because it concerns the quality of people's lives. Despite New Labour's pre-occupation with arithmetical targets, the end product of health care is not quantifiable in many instances. In reality, therefore, its performance is far more difficult to judge than many of the crude indicators to which it is subjected would suggest. To complicate things even further, the environment in which it exists is dominated not only by the interest of those it serves but also by the various professional communities that it needs in order to work smoothly (Harrison et al., 1992). These consist of a mixture of cultures that do not always see eye to eye (Harrison et al., 1992). Managers and clinicians are thus charged to adopt common goals to meet not only the short-term political agenda such as the reduction of waiting lists, but also to determine longer-term policy. In practice, the two imperatives are in conflict and NHS staff not surprisingly complain of target fatigue and low morale (Yoong and Heyman, 2003).

The specific task facing policy makers, managers and clinicians in implementing the *NHS Plan,* is to discover how best to improve access, efficiency, effectiveness and the quality of services. New Labour adopted a stance reliant on performance indicators, national standards, audit and inspection. There are, however, alternative management strategies such as allowing the diversity that is promised to primary care trusts (PCTs). Another option is competition whereby patient choice has a much bigger influence on the service. So a more modern way ahead might have sought to match central targets with a degree of local autonomy that failed to materialise thus far.

Measuring performance in the way New Labour approached this is a tricky undertaking. The standardised mortality ratio is an all-or-none indicator that is reliable. People are either alive or dead. But once there is an attempt to quantify degrees of morbidity along a continuum that moves to measure such things as quality of life, the less reliable the statistics become. Herein lies a further problem for those implementing the *NHS Plan* who are charged to measure the extent of success without any real safeguards regarding the reliability of their figures.

The *NHS Plan* was inspirational in nature and was widely approved by a wide range of both professional and lay stakeholders whose endorsement was recorded in its opening pages (DOH, 2000a). It set out a radical set of remedies for the commonly agreed deficiencies of the NHS. These can be summarised as follows:

- Low investment over decades by comparison with EU neighbours.
- Lack of national standards.
- Over-centralisation and lack of local autonomy for managers.
- Lack of clear incentives to improve performance.
- Obstacles between health and social care services and between primary and secondary care.
- Disempowered patients.
- Unnecessary demarcation between professionals.

This resulted in a massive agenda for change that can be subdivided into the following categories.

NEW FINANCIAL AND PHYSICAL INFRASTRUCTURE AND NEW SERVICES

BEDS

- 7,000 additional beds by 2004.
- 30 per cent increase in critical care beds by 2003.
- 5,000 extra intermediate care beds for the elderly.

NEW HOSPITALS

- 100 new hospitals by 2010.

NEW SERVICES

- Breast screening to be extended to women aged 70.

GENERAL TARGETS TO BE ACHIEVED BY 2004

- £1 billion investment in primary care facilities including the upgrading of 3,000 GP surgeries by 2004.
- 20 one-stop diagnostic and treatment centres for day casework.
- 400 new renal dialysis places.
- 3,000 defibrillators in public places.
- 50 new magnetic resonance imaging scanners.
- 200 new computer tomography scanners.
- 45 new linear accelerators.
- 80 liquid cytology units for cancer screening.

INFORMATION TECHNOLOGY SPENDING BY 2004

- £25 billion to connect all GPs to the NHS net, and develop electronic medical records.

STAFFING TARGETS TO BE MET BY 2004

- 7,500 additional consultant medical staff.
- 2,000 more general practitioners.

- 20,000 extra nurses.
- 6,500 more therapists.

TRAINING TARGETS BY 2004

- 100 additional medical school places.
- 5,500 nursing places.
- 4,400 therapy places.

STRONGER MANAGEMENT CONTROL LINKED TO IMPROVED EFFICIENCY

- National targets to tackle health inequalities between socio-economic groups.
- Efficiency targets to achieve common national standards in which the weakest NHS trusts were expected to match the performance of the strongest within five years.
- The establishment of a Commission for Health Improvement to co-ordinate the assessment of performance and monitor a new system of clinical governance.
- A traffic light system (that was subsequently replaced by a star rating system) to identify levels of performance on a list of common criteria.
- A National Care Standards Commission to monitor standards of care in the social care and residential sector.

SPECIFIC PERFORMANCE TARGETS BY 2004

- All patients to be able to see a health professional within 24 hours.
- All patients to access their GP within 48 hours.
- A&E attendees to be seen within four hours.

SPECIFIC PERFORMANCE TARGETS BY 2005

- All patients will be seen as part of a booked admission system.
- All out-patients to be seen within three months.
- Waiting for in-patient treatment will not exceed six months.

SPECIFIC PERFORMANCE TARGETS BY 2008

- No patient will wait longer than three months for treatment.

NEW CONTRACTS FOR DOCTORS

- GPs to be offered a Personal Medical Services Contract that will make them salaried in return for the delivery of a defined quantum of work. This will replace the General Medical Services Contract in which they have greater freedom to choose exactly what services they will offer to members of their practice panel.
- Consultants will be offered a contract that commits them more fully to the NHS and prevents new consultants engaging in private practice for the first seven years of their appointment.

NEW STRUCTURES TO ENABLE THE *PLAN* TO WORK

- A Modernisation Board comprising broad stakeholder interests and including patient's representatives to advise the secretary of state on the implementation of the *NHS Plan.*
- A Modernisation Agency that is separate from the Department of Health with a special remit to introduce the *Plan* locally. It will incorporate a number of action teams to implement the *Plan*'s prescription. Examples include the Primary Care Development Team and the Clinical Governance Support Unit.
- Task forces to enforce national policies on the reduction of targeted causes of morbidity such as heart disease and specific service-related targets such as waiting lists.
- Care trusts to be responsible for the purchase of both health care and social care in a locality.
- An NHS Leadership Centre to synchronise management and leadership development at all levels.

NEW SYSTEMS OF PROFESSIONAL REGULATION AS FOLLOWS

- UK Council for Health Regulators to oversee the work of the General Medical Council, the Nursing and Midwifery Council and the Council for the Allied Health Professions.
- Medical Education Standards Board to take the place of the individual post-graduate bodies that control the training of GPs and specialists.
- National Clinical Assessment Authority to scrutinise evidence in cases of suspected poor performance by individual medical practitioners.

NEW FORMS OF PATIENT INVOLVEMENT AS FOLLOWS

- Abolition of Community Health Councils as the official public watchdog.
- Patient Advisory and Liaison Services (PALS) to be initiated in every NHS trust to represent all aspects of patients' interests.
- Patients' Forums to be developed in every Acute Trust and PCT to bring a patient perspective to NHS planning and to the provision of services.
- A Concordat with the private sector defining the nature of outsourced, NHS funded services for such activities as elective surgery and intermediate care.

MANAGERIAL INEFFICIENCY OR TARGET FATIGUE: THE CASE OF WAITING TIMES?

As the *NHS Plan* was operationalised it soon became abundantly clear that the targets set by it and the subsequent iterations of its *Implementation Programme* were not being met, although the government reasoned to the contrary (DOH, 2000a, 2000b, 2003a; Davies, 2001). This massively detailed mega-strategy that contained over 360 targets soon began to defy the planners and perplex the managers who struggled to provide services to patients. All of this was compounded by a concurrent reorganisation of massive proportions to introduce a primary care-led service through the establishment of PCTs. These amorphous organisations that initially lacked the infrastructure necessary for their task, were intended by 2004 to purchase 75 per cent of NHS care. This therefore transferred new responsibility and its associated accountability to frontline professionals such as GPs (DOH, 2001a). The system of health service delivery began to creak under the weight of government reform, and when particular targets were not hit managers became the focus of reproach. NHS managers were reeling from target fatigue arising from the utter volume and pace of change that was expected of them.

The doyen of targets for New Labour was waiting times. The statistic can be an elusive and unreliable one. Patients can be on waiting lists unnecessarily because they fail to attend for their appointments. They move house while they are waiting and are lost from the system. They also sometimes recover spontaneously so that they do not need to take up the service that is offered, and if they die while they are waiting it can take many months to remove their name from waiting lists. Nevertheless, this is the measure that politicians believe in. It is thus used as an index of efficiency by governments in office and as a descriptor of under-funding by parties who are in opposition. The fact that some patients can afford to wait became overlooked within New Labour's passionate mission to hit waiting time targets and this led to a distortion of clinical priorities. Quite understandably, NHS trusts chose to treat those things that were easy to deal with first to reduce the total number in the queue. For instance, good results in reducing the overall number of people waiting can be achieved by intensifying investment on day case surgery rather than, say, hip replacements that are more labour intensive and generate a longer hospital stay.

Waiting times were to become the central measure of the success of the *NHS Plan* and they became connected inextricably with the blame culture that New Labour had initially aspired to eradicate. The key evidence in the story was demonstrated through the publication of various Audit Commission Reports on Waiting Times (Audit Commission, 2001, 2002, 2003a). The Audit Commission is the Government's guardian of efficiency and value for money in its public services. Its 2001 report on waiting times in A&E departments had validity and reliability in that it drew its conclusions from the replication of previous work conducted in 1996 and 1998. Its findings were critical of waiting times that had worsened nationally, and the blame for this was promptly placed on managerial shortcomings. The Commission found in mitigation, however, that the workload of A&E departments is inherently unpredictable and that managers have to strike a difficult balance between minimising waiting times and maintaining good quality care on the one hand, and avoiding over-capacity and under-occupied staff on the other.

By 2003 the problem had not gone away. Trusts were set a target to complete the initial treatment of 90 per cent of A&E attendees within four hours and their performance was to be measured over a seven-day period. Trusts invested unsustainable resources at the specified week and cancelled elective work in an attempt to meet the political target that had been set for them. An analysis of the figures showed that despite monumental effort only 30 out of 150 trusts met the requirement (Smith, 2003).

It requires only a glimmer of insight into the complexities of the service to know that waiting times are something for which no one group of staff can be made scapegoats as New Labour chose to do. Indeed it was the Department of Health itself that had invented the very targets and also that had responsibility for the system that it then opted to denigrate (Davies, 2001). A system based on clinical need rather than the ability to pay has no controls on the demands placed upon it. Inevitably, therefore, A&E departments attract patients who are not seriously ill but who nevertheless have an entitlement to a proper professional assessment. Consumers have increasingly high expectations and do not like to wait. But if the system cannot cope with the volume of users, it has to ration what it delivers and it can only do this under present policies by making patients wait. Blaming managers provides a convenient escape route. It avoids government shouldering national accountability. Furthermore, it is convenient because it was known by government spin-doctors that NHS managers are not particularly popular with the public. Criticising managers was also far easier than doing something really radical like imposing a user charge for an A&E visit that would be the most effective way to reduce unnecessary attendance.

By 2002 another example concerning waiting times arose. The length of time that patients were waiting for out-patient appointments for surgery in ear, nose and throat departments varied widely (Audit Commission, 2002). In a study using 800 cases from 10 NHS trusts, the Audit Commission found that the wait for a child needing the insertion of grommets ranged from 4 to 22 weeks; for adults having septal surgery the wait was between 9 and 70 weeks; the wait for the fitting of a hearing-aid ranged from 8 to 55 weeks. Yet waiting times were not related directly to capacity or to levels of demand and the report criticised unsystematic management and saw that as the deficiency requiring remedy rather than a need for increased resources.

The Department of Health subsequently asked the Audit Commission to make arrangements for auditors to undertake a five-year rolling programme of spot checks to reassure the public that published waiting list statistics are robust. Auditors completed 'spot checks' at 41 trusts between June and November 2002, many of them chosen because they appeared to be at risk of having errors in reporting. The methodology was designed by the Audit Commission and agreed with the Department of Health. Up to six waiting list performance indicators (PIs) were reviewed in up to five clinical specialities at each trust (Audit Commission, 2002).

There was evidence of deliberate misreporting of waiting list information at three trusts. Prompt action was taken to investigate and deal with the issues identified, including suspending staff from duty, some of whom were subsequently dismissed. In a further 19 trusts, auditors found evidence of reporting errors in at least one PI. Altogether, they found evidence of reporting errors in 30 per cent of PIs. In three trusts, the spot checks revealed no significant problems. In the other trusts, auditors considered that weaknesses in the data-collection systems increased the risk of errors in at least one PI. One trust could not provide all the information needed for the review. Waiting lists for patients with possible breast cancer were generally well managed. In most cases the level of inaccuracy was unlikely to affect the care of individual patients significantly. Trusts, however, did operate practices that are not patient-centred, offering short-notice appointments and restarting the waiting time if patients cannot attend, for example,

Spot checks provide a quick way of establishing whether there is evidence of problems in a system, such as deliberate manipulation or inadvertent errors. They can highlight areas for improvement in the management systems but cannot quantify the accuracy of waiting lists, or the overall impact on patients. Not all errors will be identified by spot checks. Most problems arose from system weaknesses caused by inadequate management arrangements for recording data and ineffective or poorly integrated IT systems. Most trusts quickly took action to improve their performance.

The Commission concluded that all NHS trusts should review their approach to collecting waiting list information drawing on the lessons of its report. These included the need for trust board-level commitment, effective procedures and training, and specifications for new IT systems that enable them to provide the required information.

The Commission believed that the Department of Health could help improve waiting list information by:

- investigating why there has been widespread misreporting, including deliberate misreporting;
- ensuring the process for patient cancellations is reasonable from the patients' perspective;
- being clear how changes in clinical practice should be reflected in waiting lists; for example, as more procedures become day cases;
- incorporating data quality standards into the control assurance framework used by trusts to manage risks.

The response of the Department of Health to this report was summarised uncompromisingly by Chief Executive Sir Nigel Crisp as follows:

> Deliberate mis-reporting of waiting list data is reprehensible and inexcusable and we have made it very clear that serious consequences will follow any individual or Trust that seek to manipulate their performance data. The code of conduct for managers sets out very clearly that it will not be tolerated. Disciplinary action has followed at the Trusts where deliberate manipulation of the figures was confirmed.
>
> Waiting lists are being replaced by computerised air-line style booking systems which will yield much more accurate and consistent data, as well as giving more choice about the times of their appointments and operation.
>
> We have already announced more than two billion [pounds] in investment to improve the IT infrastructure of the NHS. This will deliver significant benefits to managers booking patient appointments and will strengthen the data collection process. I would like all NHS Trust Chief Executives to consider the implications of the Commission's findings and review their procedures and systems to ensure that patients can have as much confidence in their data as possible. (DOH, 2003b: 1–2)

CONCLUSION

The radical reform of the NHS that commenced at the start of the 21st century was overdue and New Labour had the record budget surpluses to invest in it. It was apparent that, despite the volume of investment and unprecedented organisational change, concrete improvements were barely palpable. Certainly reforms were under way but a number of questions remain unresolved. The fundamental relationship between politicians and those delivering the service needed to change so that the direction of travel was not ideologically driven, as had been the case. Local solutions to broad targets were not being permitted and this was stifling the ingenuity that many NHS managers possess to solve problems in their own way. Although government rhetoric suggested that control was passing to frontline staff, there was still sufficient evidence of central intrusiveness into local health affairs if things were not going to plan.

There was a strong suggestion that the government could never be wrong on the NHS. It was evident from the example of meeting waiting time targets that performance management of the NHS was still confused despite the best efforts of New Labour that had become the most centralising administration in the history of the NHS. Over-regulation and the target fatigue it engendered amongst managers was a lasting issue needing to be relieved; the whole issue of the development of a more liberated and autonomous managerial cadre also needed attention. Using information to judge performance and to draw comparisons was a thoroughly reasonable objective. Yet the dubious performance indicators and methodologies in use could not justify that information being used as a blunt instrument with which to intimidate managers. A system based on fear with managers being placed on probation and having their livelihoods threatened was to become a highly dubious answer to the labyrinthine task confronting health service managers.

In its first annual report on the state of the NHS the independent watchdog, the Commission for Health Improvement (CHI), observed much on which to praise the service. But it warned that innovation and improvement was at risk because,

> The scale of organisational change in the health service which may deliver improvement in future, and the concentration on short term waiting targets, which have led to people being seen more quickly, mean that NHS leaders are very stretched 'keeping the show on the road' now, and have very limited time for other improvement activities we know can enhance services people are receiving. (CHI, 2003: 41)

Ultimately the Achilles' heel of the *NHS Plan* could also concern the massive human capital that was required to implement it fully. In 2000, the *NHS Plan* required 7,500 more consultants and 2,000 more GPs working in the NHS by 2004. In 2002, a further target was set for 15,000 more GPs and consultants to be employed within the NHS by 2008. Increasing the number of training places and poaching staff from overseas were aspects of achieving the workforce targets that were set. But maintaining morale while ever driving staff to work harder became another critical human resource management consideration, not to mention paying them enough to retain their services. General speculation suggested that these targets could take 10 years to achieve (Gray and Finlayson, 2002).

Despite the perceived shortcomings of the NHS, its popularity with users is repeatedly re-emphasised (National Centre for Social Research, 2003). The British Social Attitude Survey questioned 2,200 people on a range of social policies, including their attitudes to the NHS. Seventy-five per cent rejected private insurance solutions to its problems and favoured a publicly funded service that is universal and is free at the point of use. When the sample was broken down, support was found to be equal across the earning strata and across the main political parties. Sixty-three per cent of respondents, the highest proportion for 20 years, supported an increase in taxation for health education and welfare, and 80 per cent of these gave the NHS as their first preference thus confirming their satisfaction with the service.

The following chapter will examine the more detailed consequences of the *NHS Plan* and its subsequent iteration by identifying the salient challenges facing the NHS in the next decade.

THREE

THE MAJOR CHALLENGES FOR A MODERNISED NHS

INTRODUCTION

Despite its claims about modernisation, the *NHS Plan* can be seen as sustaining, through improved capability and additional assets, the customary NHS model that is dominated by the provision of acute care. Its blandness that its critics observed was exemplified in its recommendations for the overall public health (Calman et al., 2001). It was somewhat modest in that it failed to address initially the evidence that many causes of morbidity and mortality are beyond the scope of the NHS and reside in such diverse factors as socio-economic circumstances and personal lifestyles, something that policy makers were to recognise later (DOH, 2003d). Its targets therefore had a flavour of political pragmatism about them, notably in their pressure to get results rapidly. Certainly the *NHS Plan* was not over-emphatic on life expectancy and inequalities in life chances. It also ignored the newer concept in health research known as 'social capital' that is being used to link social support to health. Social capital is the degree of cohesion that exists in communities. It refers to processes between people that establish networks, norms and the social trust necessary to facilitate co-ordination and co-operation for the mutual benefit of citizens. This concept embodies such structures as civic and religious groups, family membership and informal networks and it bears the norms of voluntarism, altruism and trust. All of these serve to enhance the benefits of investment for better health that are thought to correlate positively with improved health status such as increased life expectancy and reduced infant mortality (WHO, 1998). The *NHS Plan* assumed originally, however, that the NHS is capable of achieving optimum end results in isolation. Yet in reality, the multifactorial origins of many causes of ill health to which this ground-breaking new policy drew attention, require far more substantial social engineering and a cross-disciplinary approach involving several government departments as well as the strategic involvement of local government and a whole host of other community-based resources.

That said, the *NHS Plan* contained much that was well intended. But for its successful implementation, four major key factors require close consideration. These are:

- the decentralisation of authority;
- the leadership conundrum;
- the patient as a consumer;
- patient choice and the role of competition.

THE DECENTRALISATION OF AUTHORITY

As has been demonstrated in Chapter 2 (page 40), in the case of waiting times there has been a dogmatic firmness from central government on meeting political targets irrespective of whether these coincide with the priorities of particular local communities. All of this gives way to a short-termist mentality that can contain quite perverse expectations. Although the *NHS Plan* made reference to what it called 'earned autonomy', this had not meant that managers were free from an over-abundance of inspections, audits and a requirement to meet multiple performance targets simultaneously. The whole approach could be seen to work on the faulty machine model. By viewing the service as a machine, government sustained a belief that reducing variation in the performance of its systemic components would improve its overall organisational performance. This emphasis on the controls that were wielded by NHS leaders ignored theories that suggest that managerial creativity comes from facilitation rather than dogmatism wherein a certain amount of general direction is accompanied by freedoms for managers to exercise some personal discretion and flair (Plsek and Wilson, 2001). Yet central command and control in the NHS is such that it even takes trouble to dictate the obvious things that Florence Nightingale could have told us: for example, that hospitals should be kept clean and that patients should have nourishing food. All of this generates mistrust whereby managers and individuals are kept looking over their shoulder for the next burst of ministerial engagement. In reaction to this, there arose authoritative calls for the NHS to be de-politicised and for a clearer separation between government and the delivery of health care (Kings Fund, 2002). This would enable service managers to manage their own affairs while still conforming to a set of standards that are set independently of government. This, it was believed, would increase the sense of local ownership of the NHS without sacrificing its public accountability.

Any reservations about the limitations of the *NHS Plan* with regard to the distribution of authority within the NHS were alleviated somewhat in the year following its publication (DOH, 2001a). Frontline staff were to be given a significant stake in the balance of power when 75 per cent of spending decisions were to be determined by primary care trusts (PCTs) from 2004. It has been suggested that this is calculated to extract the traditional control from secondary care providers and to transfer it to PCTs (Calman et al., 2001). But this was not without risk given the infancy of PCTs and their lack of experience in financial transactions of the magnitude that were to be expected of them. It seemed probable also, that the success in terms of the overall public health would depend on GPs accepting a form of the then Personal Medical Services Contract. This would reduce their freedoms as independent contractors and provide financial incentives for them to provide a range of services tailored more specifically to the needs of their practice populations.

THE LEADERSHIP CONUNDRUM

The devolution of power is inseparable from the issue of leadership, and indeed the repeated criticism of managerial inadequacies of NHS managers by health ministers came as something of a paradox in that it was in conflict with what has been said elsewhere by New Labour. The Cabinet Office Performance and Innovation Unit recognised in a far-reaching report that Britain's public services face unprecedented challenges at the start of the 21st century (Cabinet Office, 2001). The report openly acknowledged the need to modernise public services like the NHS and orient them more closely towards the needs, wishes and higher expectations of the general public, and it advocated for partnerships both across the public sector and with private and voluntary organisations.

The Cabinet Office report recognised that there was much outstanding leadership in the public services. But it also pointed to evidence suggesting that the public services were not attracting or keeping the best leaders and that they did not have sufficiently robust strategies for recruiting high quality talent to the posts that are most crucial. The Commission for Health Improvement also went on to endorse this observation (CHI, 2003). It noted the overall difficulty of getting the best people in key places and it claimed also that the general quality of leadership in the NHS was weakened, in particular, by the reluctance of doctors to take up leadership positions.

The Cabinet Office report thus accepted generally that jobs and careers in services such as the NHS attract little in the way of plaudits and that top management jobs are probably underpaid in relation to the responsibilities that the post holders shoulder. While there were many leadership development initiatives, including the NHS Leadership Centre, there was little verification of their effectiveness. The Cabinet Office, unlike its health ministers, recognised that public service leaders were often unable to lead effectively because others deny them the autonomy, the backing, or even to undertake the challenges that enable them to do so.

It seemed somewhat curious to the reporters that there was little shared understanding of the qualities required for effective leadership in the NHS. While personal qualities were thought important, ministers have tended to have these overridden by doctrinaire policies that were shackling initiative. Not surprisingly, therefore, NHS managers themselves were often unable to account personally for their own success or for the lack of it. What was seemingly missing was a better balance between the liberty to lead and the overriding accountability for hitting political performance targets.

What seems fundamental to improved leadership in the NHS, therefore, is an improved and shared understanding about what is feasible. Acknowledging openly that some NHS trusts just do not have the capacity to accomplish all that is required of them is a mature thing to do and prevents individuals and organisations being set up to fail. This would do much to alleviate the blame culture that had prevailed. Poor performing trusts with perceived weak leadership were being put out to franchise and enigmatic managerial supremos, who have been successful elsewhere, were intended to be brought in to replace the existing management that was to be summarily removed. It could be argued that this served only to generate uncertainty and fear and took the chance of creating an obedient managerial class that is risk averse and reluctant to question government dogma, let alone answer back.

The Cabinet Office report admitted that the government must offer a better deal for public service leaders to make the public sector more enticing (Cabinet Office, 2001). This, it believed, should offer attractive careers that value proficiency and encourage innovative leadership roles. It concluded that:

Public service leaders require appropriate challenge from those to whom they are accountable (politicians, non-executives and inspectorates). But they also need to be given the space in which to lead from politicians and central government. Policy-makers should more systematically take account of the effects of policies, guidance and legislation in either encouraging or constraining leadership. Departments should ensure that relations between politicians and chief executives are clarified and promote initiatives in joint training of political and administrative leaders. Inspection bodies should collectively look at leadership performance. (Cabinet Office, 2001, Executive Summary: 3–4)

This highly rational set of observations was slow to penetrate the NHS where politicians have often intervened in local NHS managerial affairs as though they *are* the managers.

Besides having been examined from a position of political pragmatism, NHS management has been studied at a more analytical level. In a study of managers at every level of the service and through attendance at many meetings, biting criticism of NHS management was made by Sergeant (2003). This work found deficiencies at top management level, where it was claimed managers lacked the basic tools to do the job. The researcher observed that, 'Chief Executives cannot reward the excellent. Nor can they sack the incompetent (or not without difficulty)' (Sergeant, 2003: 5).

Chief executives were overburdened by political targets, and middle managers were pressurised constantly to provide information to the Department of Health. Even at the front line, ward managers felt a similar weight of bureaucracy and the anger of consultants at all of this, was a further prominent finding within the work of Sergeant. As in similar studies, the solution was seen in giving managers the freedom, authority and financial control to manage in a way that gives direction to local circumstances.

THE PATIENT AS A CONSUMER

The participation of health service users can be viewed on two levels, as outlined below.

INTERPERSONAL PARTICIPATION

Recent times have seen a sea change in the direct practice of health care that is partly a response to rising public expectations. Indeed, some quite fundamental philosophical developments have occurred concerning a new emphasis on patient involvement in the more enlightened parts of the NHS. These have required significant cultural changes that are intended to transform the traditional role of the patient as a passive recipient of health care to a more inclusive position that encourages patient participation (DOH, 1998a, 2000b, 2000c, 2002d).

Conventional definitions of professionalism and their associated masculine perspectives emphasise the promotion of rational, objective and formal knowledge and place health professionals in a privileged position of power over the service user (Wilkins, 2000). Indeed, there is a long history of authoritarianism within health care professional circles and it is interesting to consider from where this power emanated. On the one hand, it could be argued that it derived from a transparent and sound scientific professional basis, whilst on the other hand, some argue that it arose as a result of the mystique associated with professional knowledge and skills (Ellis, 1988).

Professionals are not unaware of the inequalities between themselves and patients and some seek actively to alleviate powerlessness, ignorance and dependence. Similarly, some patients will be reluctant to express a preference because they see the doctor, nurse, midwife and therapist as the expert. So mutuality is a complex matter and few professionals have created an alliance that puts patients on equal terms with them. The rationale for securing greater participation accepts that the professionals have a more expert but general knowledge of health and illness and its management. But it also recognises that patients have a personal experience of these factors because only they know their own feelings, social circumstances, habits, attitudes to risk, values and preferences. Both types of knowledge are needed, therefore, to administer care and treatment successfully with the open recognition that patients can also possess vital expertise. Acknowledging that element of personal knowledge allows patients to share responsibility for their care and to be offered rational, practical choices that remove the time-honoured expectation of acquiescence.

The anticipation that patient preferences will become the norm is a challenge for professionals (Say and Thomson, 2003). It embodied practical considerations such as extra consulting time and difficulties in finding out what patients might prefer. Health professionals have not been trained in the approach so there is a demand on their capability. Furthermore, if patients' preferences contradict those of the professionals what then is to be done?

Unashamed consumerism in its generally accepted sense is probably not a feasible option for the NHS but an appreciation that the professional does not always know best provides a recipe for the coalition that policies are attempting to secure. This reinforces the view that patients are equals with different expertise to that of the professionals which implies the sharing of power (Coulter, 2002). It therefore constitutes a non-hierarchical association based on trust and mutual respect for each other's contribution (Hunt and Symonds, 1995).

POLITICAL AND POLICY INVOLVEMENT

The idea of consumerism in relation to the politics of health and of health policy is also not new to the NHS. Attempts have been made for some time to listen to the users of its services (Cox et al., 1993). Yet the political interpretation of consumerism has shifted over the last two decades.

Initially there was a collectivist approach to the service user whereby Community Health Councils allegedly represented a broad range of community interests. The modern, seemingly more personalised, approach goes farther and seeks the political representation of the individual patient (DOH, 1998a, 2002d). Endeavours now centre on the empowerment of users of services by actively involving them in decision making at all levels of policy making, planning and care delivery (DOH, 2002d). Whereas the previous arrangements kept users at a distance by attempting mainly to respond to their observations, the new model embraces them as part of the NHS and provides a platform from which they can comment upon, influence and thus shape current and future services (Higgins, 1993; Blaxter, 1995; DOH, 2002d).

This is in stark contrast to the very passive role for patients associated with the historical interpretation of consumer involvement in the NHS. The introduction of this new government strategy is simply a starting point, but what has proved elusive is the capture of the genuine representativeness of all consumers because the views of many of them are so elusive. This remains an inherent feature of current policy, which is more emphatic than ever that the voice of the patient should be at the heart of the NHS (DOH, 2002d). These contemporary pronouncements express explicit intentions to increase patient choice and go so far as to assert that, 'further steps will change the relationship between patients and services. Patients will be in the driving seat' (DOH, 2002d: 24).

This new political attitude to consumerism has also produced a shift in the overall organisational culture of the NHS. Attempts are thus being made not solely to allay discontent with the service but to match the expectations of patients. This movement has been described as making the 'invisible hospital' visible to the users and to juxtapose more closely the world of the patient with that of the professional (Spiers, 1995). The dissonance between the professional and the lay user of health services is a topic much debated in the literature. But with this new alliance comes a repositioning of the service user as a significant player in the determination of the level, nature and standard of services and as a full participant in the planning as well as being a recipient of NHS services. Despite the espoused ambitions of New Labour to involve users, knowing how, when and where to involve them and how to prepare staff for the users' new role remains unresolved.

The New Labour government established, in January 2003, a Commission for Patient and Public Involvement in Health for which legislation was needed. This abolished Community Health Councils in late 2003. The Commission's membership is designed to oversee an elaborate framework of Change Assessment Groups at Strategic Health Authority level and Patient Advocacy Forums at each NHS trust with new powers of inspection and representation on trust boards (DOH, 2002d). This commitment to improving the patient experience concerns what New Labour has referred to as 'putting the patient at the centre of the NHS', and this serves to highlight how patient and public involvement can impact on local health services (DOH, 2003e).

PCTs are required to produce a prospectus aimed at informing the public and patients about health services in their area. These documents contain information about local services, including:

- the results of an annual survey of patients within local trusts and the action taken subsequently;
- a breakdown of how the local NHS budget is spent;
- performance assessment ratings;
- planned improvements to local services;
- useful contact details and numbers.

These arrangements look to address the democratic deficit in local NHS accountability. Democratically elected local government Overview and Scrutiny Committees (OSCs) are intended to scrutinise substantial variations and developments in local NHS service provision. The powers for OSCs came into force in January 2003 and their impact was intended to be felt increasingly. The task of OSCs is to decide which areas of the NHS they wish to scrutinise. The power of overview and scrutiny of health services builds upon the existing powers of local authorities to promote social, economic and environmental well-being. This creates a new role for elected councillors as community leaders. Supporting the health scrutiny powers are three key duties that were placed on the NHS, thus:

- NHS bodies must consult OSCs on any substantial development or variation that it intends to introduce;
- NHS bodies must provide information about services and decisions affecting services;
- senior officers of NHS bodies must attend OSC meetings to answer questions.

As the statutory consultee for major changes to the NHS, OSCs have the power of referral to the secretary of state where they may contest a proposal both on the grounds of inadequate consultation or if they believe that the proposal is not in the interests of local people.

From April 2003 every NHS trust and PCT established a Patient Advice and Liaison Service (PALS) to provide on-the-spot help, support and information to patients, their families and carers. PALS also began to provide valuable, local feedback to trusts on what people are saying to enable them to respond positively and change services to better meet the needs of the people who use them.

Section 11 of the Health and Social Care Act 2001 was implemented in January 2003 and it brought to NHS organisations a legal requirement that they must consult and involve patients and the public in several ways. These were as follows:

- not just when a major change is proposed, but in the ongoing planning of services;
- not solely when considering a proposal but in developing that proposal;
- on decisions that may affect the operation of services.

New Labour's plans are complemented by an undeniable appetite for information among patients and those who use services; the Cochrane Consumer Collaboration Network (www.cochraneconsumer.com/) is but one source of valuable information that is available to them. This intends to be comprehensible and relatively free from technical language and to provide user-friendly information. A respectable literature is also beginning to be assembled to describe the techniques available to consumers when they search for health-related information on the internet (Eysenbach and Kohler, 2002).

Policy strives to achieve greater accountability from the NHS but the extent to which consumer involvement is feasible or desirable provokes a varied response. At a theoretical level, there is debate about the appropriateness of the very idea that consumers of NHS services are in any way comparable to consumers in a free-market economy (Blaxter, 1995). Consumerism implies rational choices based on information with the ability to evaluate the alternative options that are available. Arguably, therefore, NHS users are in a vastly different position than they are, for example, when they purchase consumer goods, for several reasons. NHS users find themselves located within a service that has finite resources and this means that choice will always be restricted. While they might be increasingly well informed, there is an inevitable disparity between the technical knowledge possessed by them and that available to the professionals who are managing their care. This has led to an entrenched 'in-house' convention among the more rigid professionals. They argue that clinical decisions, care and treatment cannot be seen to be consumer services in the way that, for instance, hotel or catering services in the NHS might be judged and that the former are not really the business of the patient.

Being a partner relies on professionals being willing to share knowledge and it has been argued that partnership does not necessarily confer empowerment (Lamont, 1999). For the detractors from the consumer empowerment of patients, therefore, the intention to involve patients is something that could be somewhat cosmetic because, although laudable entirely in its intent, the reality is that some professionals are conditioned socially not to relinquish their power. True participation relies on more than being heard and has to get beyond mere consultation if it is to be effective.

It has been contended that to treat patients as equals is false democracy, with the comment that:

> Denial of the status of doctors and of medicine's tradition of research is false democracy. It is an attempt to avoid destructive envy. Destructive envy denigrates and spoils that which is needed, biting the hand that feeds us or cutting off one's nose to spite one's face. More than other professional groups, doctors are envied. Partly this derives from the inequality of the relationship between doctors and patients. (McQueen, 2002: 1214)

PATIENT CHOICE AND THE ROLE OF COMPETITION

CHOICE

At the inception of the NHS, expectations were low, deference to professionals was the norm and there was an overall indifference to patients on the part of policy makers. New Labour attempted through its ambitious *NHS Plan* to reverse this trend by providing services that are responsive to individual need. In New Labour's first term of office from 1997–2001 it introduced top-down reforms through the creation of service targets, inspection regimes and national standards. This national framework of standards was important to improve geographical equity. In its second term from 2001, however, it left these structures in place but introduced change that was intended to work from the bottom upwards (Milburn, 2003). The decisive elements of its intended reform programme were to become:

- The decentralisation of commissioning to PCTs to meet the needs of local communities.
- The creation of NHS foundation trusts to free them from bureaucracy and entrust them to the hands of local people.
- The encouragement of a range of different providers of services to NHS patients that used public, private and voluntary providers, any of whom were to meet commonly agreed standards and be subject to a common system of inspection.

These reforms aimed to extend choices for patients. No health care system can provide unlimited choice and indeed most private health insurance schemes in the UK exclude maternity care, primary care, psychiatric and other chronic degenerative conditions. So there was an acknowledgement that there are limits to choice in the NHS because about a third of what it does has some urgency attached to it where time is of the essence (Milburn, 2003). Nevertheless, sufficient of the NHS is planned in advance to both introduce and to expand choices, especially for procedures that are elective. Examples include:

- Choices in maternity care, between a midwife-led service and a consultant-led one, between a birth at home and one in hospital.
- Choice in the selection of a family doctor and through a GP, to book the time of hospital appointments that are convenient to the patient.
- The option for patients requiring coronary bypass surgery who have waited over six months to be treated in an alternative to their local hospital in either the NHS or private sector.
- Patients waiting for a cataract operation in London who have waited over six months at one hospital can be offered an alternative hospital.
- From summer 2003 patients in London waiting more than six months for any form of elective surgery were offered the choice of an alternative hospital.
- From summer 2003 in Greater Manchester those needing orthopaedic, ENT and general surgery will also be offered choice if they have been waiting longer than six months.
- From summer 2004 all patients waiting six months for any form of elective surgery will be able to choose at least one alternative hospital and normally four, be they public or private hospitals.
- From December 2005 choice will be extended from those patients waiting longest for hospital treatment to *all* patients. Those needing elective surgery will be able to select from at least four or five different hospitals, including both NHS and private sector providers.
- Beyond 2005, patients needing surgery will be able to choose from more hospitals in which they can be treated.
- In primary care the role of pharmacists in disease management will increase. More drugs will be sold over the counter rather than needing a doctor's prescription.
- NHS Direct will be extended and more NHS walk-in centres created.
- A specialist GP will see patients who have been referred ordinarily to hospital for minor surgery or for out-patient consultations locally.

The biggest threat to choice in the NHS is the limits imposed by the volume of patients it can accommodate at any one time. The service has to deal at times with quite unpredictable demands on it and this means that its facilities become unavoidably stretched. New Labour's investment plan attempted to deal with this through novel solutions such as maximising capacity in its own premises and by purchasing spare capacity from the private sector. The concept of the diagnostic and treatment centres was planned to be available to 250,000 patients a year by 2005 to focus on elective surgery in the NHS and by private sector providers. New private sector developments were to be encouraged and a concordat to expand the relationship between the NHS and the voluntary sector was signed (DOH, 2000d).

A case against offering choice, however, concerns equity. For instance, giving choice to one patient for, say, an expensive treatment might mean that another is treated with a cheaper remedy or has to wait and is thus treated less fairly. What is certain is that services are not spread evenly and this is demonstrated by the variation in waiting times nationally for identical episodes of treatment. This means there are inequities in the availability of treatment that necessarily curtails choice between providers. Furthermore, there are inequities in outcomes for patients and this is demonstrated in high-profile cases where adverse events occur. Inequity can also be seen in the disparity of mortality and morbidity rates among the lower socio-economic groups. In reality, therefore, choice has mainly been available previously for those with the ability to buy priority through private health care. Buying care privately is also somewhat illusory because the selfsame NHS consultants treat private patients, in either NHS facilities or in private hospitals. This means that the preferential treatment they buy comprises convenience, privacy and better hotel facilities rather than better technical care.

A further debate concerns the ability of the majority of the public to exercise choice in what are often very sophisticated matters in which sometimes there are no options. In reality, choice will not be from a range of alternatives; rather it will be between different suppliers of the same service (Appleby et al., 2003). New Labour's progressive thinking assumed optimistically, however, that the NHS should plan for an information age where most people will be well informed and will not only want choices but will demand to exercise them. Like the previous Conservative government, therefore, New Labour's policy on choice was an example that the state paternalism that characterised the post-war welfare state is being eroded.

During the Conservative years the uptake of private insurance was used as an index of dissatisfaction with the NHS. The more people that entered into private insurance subscriptions, the worse the NHS was claimed to be performing. The corollary for a high level of insurance uptake is that the NHS needs to exist solely for the less well-off and then it would only need to meet minimum standards. Extended choice, however, is expected to reassure the public and discourage them from opting out of the NHS. To this end patients will be helped to make informed choices through easily obtainable information on hospital performance, quality and waiting times, all of which seems a tall order given that so little information of this type is generated for the use of patients. To enhance choice depends therefore on better administrative information, and the electronic booking of hospital appointments from the GP surgery became a target for all parts of the NHS by December 2005.

The medical profession is particularly sceptical that patients can be consumers and should have unlimited choice and an unbridled access to information. The views of those doctors who are most antagonistic can be summarised as follows:

> As an increasing number of patients demand their rights the NHS struggles to meet these demands. Staff feel that they cannot keep up with rising expectations ... the choice facing the government and the media is stark: either engage in a meaningful debate over the scope of the NHS or the organisation will crumple. (Wardrope, 2002: 1369)

COMPETITION

Extending choices to patients that are linked to the payment for services that they bring with them renders them the essential economic unit within health care financial transactions, and means that NHS providers will then have to compete for patients. Such a system carries with it the unambiguous incentive to providers of attracting as many patients as possible. A system of payment by results in which resources will follow the choices patients make has the potential to define an increasing proportion of each hospital's income. The key organisations in the delivery of this choice-driven system are PCTs and NHS foundation hospitals. This system requires NHS foundation trusts to improve their efficiency and their standards in ways that improve both their functioning as well as adding to the quality of the care that patients receive. Securing patient satisfaction is a principal objective of offering greater choice. Yet while this is primarily about improving the patient's lot, it does (in theory) give them more power and influence once they are able to decide where, so to speak, to place their business.

The creation of NHS foundation hospital trusts is at the heart of the debate concerning competition and their creation fuelled considerable political controversy. This arose initially from academic sources that questioned the logic underpinning the entire idea (Robinson, 2002; Klein, 2003). Ideological opponents followed it swiftly from within the Labour Party and the trade union movement were also vociferously opposed to what they saw to be an idea that might well have originated in the Conservative Party (Kmietowicz, 2002; UNISON, 2003). The premise on which NHS foundation hospitals were conceived concerned their social ownership. The presumption, therefore, was that their control would pass to the local community and out of the hands of central government. These organisations were intended to behave as competing mutual societies that were to be introduced incrementally over about a five-year period commencing in 2003. The extent of their freedoms did, however, become a matter for intense debate.

Superficially, NHS foundation hospital trusts could be viewed as a staging post for privatising the NHS. This suspicion was intensified when not only existing trusts were allowed to become NHS foundation trusts but also other organisations from the private or voluntary sectors were invited to seek foundation status. On the other hand, there were levels of regulation intended to keep them as part of the NHS family, although these were not without ambiguity (DOH, 2002c).

Criticism that foundation trusts would not lead to greater local accountability or social ownership also arose. As public services, the public as a whole already owned NHS hospitals. In contrast, the principles on which mutual societies operate are for the benefit of their 'members'. This raised additional questions about the role of the proposed regulator, the relationship between that office and other regulatory bodies such as the Commission for Health Audit and Inspection (CHAI) with inspectorial powers over foundation trusts. It provoked further doubt from its critics about the whole political nature of the office of the regulator given that the secretary of state was still to be answerable to parliament on the NHS. They alleged that the regulator would be nothing other than a mouthpiece for the secretary of state, thus making the whole exercise in the devolution of power nothing short of a mirage. The position was summarised as follows:

> Not only do the governance arrangements of individual foundation trusts need to be sorted out, but so, most crucially, does the role of the independent regulator who is to be accountable to parliament through the secretary of state. Will he or she be the secretary of state's creature or act as a baffle, protecting foundation trusts from political intervention? Who will answer questions from members of parliament and who will react to newspaper headlines if not the minister's private office? (Klein, 2003: 175)

The introduction of the idea of foundation hospitals also brought fears that the NHS would become a two-tier service with big differences in opportunity between NHS trusts that received foundation status first and those that were at the end of the queue. It was predicted that NHS foundation trusts would enjoy greater freedom than other NHS trusts over asset disposals and financial surpluses that they would be able to keep (Kmietowicz, 2002; UNISON, 2003). New Labour parried the accusation by pledging decisively that no NHS trust would be left behind and promptly created a 'help fund' for weaker trusts and pledged that all would have foundation status by 2008 (DOH, 2003f).

Suspicion was also aroused that foundation trusts would inevitably open up a competitive commercial market into the NHS. Under this market, PCTs would commission services from a range of different providers across the public and private sectors. Providers would obviously compete for business and would pursue the most lucrative patients. It was believed that foundation trusts would have such power that weaker providers would be compelled to close non-profitable services to stay viable or run the risk of going out of business (UNISON, 2003).

The issue of value for money was a further concern because of the freedom of foundation trusts to borrow from the private sector to fund capital developments. It was feared that this would incur higher interest rates than if they were to borrow through the public sector. It was believed also that this would take them out of Treasury control but still leave them as a liability to the taxpayer if they were to get into financial difficulties.

NHS foundation trusts were also to have freedoms to set their own pay and conditions of service for staff. This aroused misgivings that they would destabilise the local health economy by drawing scarce staff away from trusts that did not have foundation status and so compound their existing staff recruitment and retention problems.

Lastly, the critics of foundation trusts feared the undermining of the principles of public service on which the NHS operates. This was typified by the recommendations of the House of Commons Health Select Committee. In a report that culminated in 39 detailed recommendations, which was based on extensive oral evidence from a broad constituency of sources, it cast serious doubts on the entire idea of foundation status (Health Select Committee, 2003). It doubted the preparedness of most NHS trust hospitals to assume the level of responsibility they were to be given and warned of the excessive bureaucracy that would flow from the intended arrangements to make NHS foundation trusts accountable to the public. It too was especially vehement of the proposed local accountability arrangements, suggesting that this would raise expectations of the NHS within local communities that were unlikely to be met. The Committee predicted that aggressive poaching of staff by NHS foundation trusts would occur, resulting in wage inflation. It contended that health care requires careful inter-agency collaboration and co-ordination and it also claimed that as weaker performing hospitals lost their best staff, their performance would deteriorate resulting in a second-class service. The existence of independent NHS foundation trusts was thought to be capable of creating the entrepreneurial behaviour that would build institutional barriers and become a hindrance to service planning as well as to the provision of seamless care to individuals. Its summary judgements were that foundation hospitals would lead to a service that was fragmented, confusing and inequitable. The strength of concern of the opponents of foundation hospitals had considerable repercussions politically, and the Health and Social Care Bill was defeated in the House of Lords in late 2003. The New Labour government invoked the Parliament Bill that effectively overturned the decision of their Lordships and brought the enabling legislation back to the Commons. Following a rancorous debate it was passed by a majority of just 17 votes in a Parliament in which New Labour had a majority of 160, and its enactment was in no small measure due to Northern Ireland and Scottish Labour MPs whose countries were not even subject to its consequences.

IS THE NHS REALLY IMPROVING?

An independently commissioned report on behalf of the Nuffield Trust considered that, at a conservative estimate, between 1999 and 2003, £835 million was spent on initiatives to improve quality in the NHS (Leatherman, 2003). This work produced a mid-term evaluation of New Labour's health reforms. It used interview data from senior NHS professionals and experts in examining access to care, its effectiveness, organisational capacity, public perceptions and variations in equity of provision. The research studied the conceptual basis for current policy initiatives and found that considerable palpable improvement was in evidence and that there was further potential for the quality to improve still further. The report identified the strengths of the service and its weaknesses, which resided in its own self-evaluation techniques and were observed to be under-developed, relative to the volume of innovation that was originating from policies. In part, this was attributable to the Department of Health's role as purchaser, provider and regulator, tasks that contained mutual contradictions. The main recommendations of the work were that professionals and patients had a bigger role in evaluation and that the establishment of a formal National Quality Information Centre was needed to systematically establish and to properly recognise the extent of achievement that was occurring.

The *NHS Plan* overtly attempts to increase capability by building new facilities and by giving new incentives to providers to attract and treat more patients and to treat them more rapidly than ever before (DOH, 2000a). It has been seen that a plurality of provision is also being encouraged (DOH, 2002b). This is intended to introduce innovation and new ways of working from a bigger array of providers, with the resulting competition inducing better performance. The likely success of achieving these things is unpredictable, but from an optimistic perspective this has been described as follows:

Only time will tell. But if the airline business is anything to go by, things will certainly be different, and the cosy duopoly of NHS and mainstream private providers will be a thing of the past. (Dash, 2004: 342)

CONCLUSION

Government became unequivocal about the successful implementation of the *NHS Plan*. It cited its achievements as follows (DOH, 2003g):

- improved access and quality of services had occurred;
- increased investment for the future was being made;
- guarantees that pay levels were sufficient to attract and retain staff had been prepared;
- unavoidable cost increases were to be met, such as inflation on goods and services.

In organisational terms the structural changes that have been introduced were not without risk. GPs selected their careers often because they sought a degree of independence and freedom from the organisational structures and hierarchies in secondary care. At the time of the introduction of the *NHS Plan*, most GPs are effectively independent contractors. Under the PCT arrangements they were becoming both managers and managed and this was something for which they were hardly trained. They were being given the spending power that can extract control from hospital consultants in a serious way if they chose to use it. Accepting new ways of team working that required vast inter-agency co-operation would similarly be needed and this was also foreign to many GP practices.

NHS foundation trusts added to what is an organisationally complicated NHS. Their creation restated the prominence of acute care and produces a distraction from the intention to produce a primary care-led service. In addition, the freedoms and investment given to foundation trusts added to the fragmentation of the service and risked making it more difficult for less well-endowed weaker trusts to improve their performance. By contrast, their potency could be a source of major organisational transformation. The NHS had been subjected to a style of command and control that was unrivalled in any government service other than the military. So NHS foundation trusts might just provide an imaginative alternative. What their detractors feared was that their freedoms would not render them answerable to the public or to the taxpayer rather than the alternative sympathies that supported their release of the current ministerial stranglehold (Walshe, 2003).

For the first time in over 50 years it was recognised through the *NHS Plan* that patients will never get a good deal out of the NHS while they are totally disempowered. The real extent of patient choice that is feasible, however, remains uncertain. Regarding patients as citizens rather than subjects should change their status and support partnership relationships with them. This could place patients at the hub of the NHS services. Idealistic though this is, it does not address professional cultures that are very adept at disempowering patients. Furthermore, the resources of the NHS are finite and this puts automatic constraints on what it can afford. So while patients appear to be given power through choice it seems highly unlikely that their GP will not act for them in almost all instances.

The NHS is unique among health systems internationally. No other Western country has a central command-and-control health system that is funded almost entirely from general taxation. Keeping an NHS in its current form and rendering it affordable is the critical issue. The *NHS Plan* was launched and began to be implemented when the economy was strong. Its prognostications rely on this remaining the case. It is also reliant on the demands of other spending ministries remaining stable, such as education, transport and defence. Other similar nations also supplement the state's contribution to health care with other funding inputs such as user payments and social insurance. These alternative sources of funding and ways of optimising the use of existing funds will form the focus of the next chapter.

FOUR

GENERATING FINANCIAL RESOURCES AND MAKING BETTER USE OF THEM

INTRODUCTION

Reference was made in Chapter 2 (page 29) to the equity principles on which the NHS was founded and to the ways in which government have adhered to these. Indeed, it is these same principles that underpinned the *NHS Plan* that was New Labour's 10-year scheme for modernisation, considered in Chapter 3 (page 46) (DOH, 2000a).

It is these objectives concerning fairness within the NHS that also form the kernel of the debate about how it should be funded so that these can be met adequately. Equity in British health care concerns care and treatment that is:

- largely free at the point of delivery;
- comprehensive in its range of services;
- available when it is needed and is based on clinical priority rather than the ability to pay;
- of a consistent standard that confers equality of clinical outcomes irrespective of the locality where treatment is provided;
- non-discriminatory in terms of age, gender, ethnicity or disability.

All governments of whatever political persuasion have signed up to these admirable intentions that have set a time-honoured culture and operational philosophy for the NHS and for its staff. Yet all governments have recognised tacitly that meeting all of these most laudable of intentions is unachievable in practice and it is the idealistic nature of these aspirations that is at the heart of the funding problems of the NHS and that confront any political administration, chancellor or health secretary. In reality, there is persistent friction between equity and efficiency (Sassi et al., 2001). In trying to treat one person fairly, resources are denied to someone else. For instance, health promotion aimed at reducing heart disease among lower socio-economic classes is an undisputed equity target. Yet in pursuing it, resources might be spent less efficiently than if they were directed at therapeutic treatment of those from the same population group who have existing heart disease.

THE CAUSES OF FUNDING PRESSURES IN BRITISH HEALTH CARE

The NHS is an inevitable victim of its own success. This is epitomised by New Labour policies to employ more doctors, nurses and therapists to move patients through the system more rapidly. This has obvious implications for the salary bill, and the increased activity also impacts to the cost of treatments. Greater investment in information technology and improvements in care quality are similarly illustrative of more work and treating more patients increasing strain on the available funds.

The NHS has 1.3 million employees and is the biggest employer in Europe and, in consequence, its wage costs are able to consume over 75 per cent of its income so that makes pay bargaining a principal component of its financial management strategy (Morris, 2003). This in turn exacerbates the political problems for government if it is always seen to be in dispute over pay with one key group of staff or another.

The continuing debate about scarce resources and rationing in the NHS confirm that both the causes of its other main demand-side problems and the solutions to them are largely self-evident. The pressure on resources comes primarily from the effects on health spending emanating from an escalating elderly population that will increase substantially over the next 30 years. The older people become the more they tend to use the NHS, and this is exemplified by a year-on-year increase in the number of prescriptions they receive (DOH, 2002e).

The other unavoidable pressure on funding arises from novel technological improvements that can be more costly than the procedures they replace. There are some exceptions to this rule with the most modern exception being micro-surgery. In the past, if a new drug or a new piece of equipment became available it would be pressed unquestioningly into use with only scant consideration for how effective it might be. Currently, however, rigorous cost–benefit evaluation of new technologies and drugs by the National Institute for Clinical Excellence is the norm so that it becomes possible to invest only in those innovations that produce the most cost-effective results. Again, this leaves government politically vulnerable if it is seen to be denying to particular patients, some treatment that, though available, is not thought to be good value for money.

Reorganisations of the health service and the administrative and bureaucratic consequences of specific government policies and the targets that it sets are another source of expenditure that is difficult to measure. These often go largely unquantified, especially if they seem more bureaucratic than what preceded them and they are liable therefore to carry a political risk to the government of the day.

SETTING THE BUDGET

Observers of the NHS are unanimous that the ability to fund the elaborate nature of the overall grand plan is at the core of its financial dilemmas simply because the nation has exceeded its capacity to afford all of the care and treatment that is available to it. The NHS has never had funding cuts, but it has experienced low growth. Governments are always proud of the increased *total* resource that they have committed to health spending year on year. This certainly has permitted a health service that has become massively more productive in terms of the numbers of patients treated, and also in the improved quality of the care and treatment that they receive. Yet in analysing the genuine level of investment made, there needs to be some discrimination between *total* growth and *real* growth. Real growth is the true amount of money available to be spent on patient care when factors such as pay increases for staff, increased employer national insurance contributions, overall inflationary pressures and the increasing costs of key supplies such as pharmaceuticals are taken into account. It will be seen as the chapter progresses that New Labour invested unprecedented new money in the NHS in the early 21st century, yet there remained reports well into its second term in office that one in seven NHS trusts was facing severe financial difficulties (NAO, 2003a). Compensatory investment that is directed at the problems of the NHS is not necessarily a panacea and this is illustrated by the failure to solve waiting list problems (discussed in Chapter 2 on page 40) because new money is apt to disappear down a 'black hole'. It follows, therefore, that there is no automatic agreement among the major political parties about either the appropriate level of NHS funding at any particular time or by what means this should be raised. So with almost sequential regularity, any vested interest that chooses is able to claim that the NHS is in permanent penury. What is non-controversial is that the demands upon what has to be a finite resource are actually infinite.

Any attempt to predict the NHS budget is clearly a precarious matter. For despite having a sound grasp of the foreseeable causes of demand there are many unpredictable occurrences that can arise within any particular fiscal year. For instance, the outbreak of a new epidemic of an infectious disease can divert resources away from their intended destination and can be impossible to anticipate. It could be expected that economic decisions are the main determinants of the actual allocation to the NHS by the Treasury each year. While this seems a reasonably systematic, technical matter, the politicised nature of the NHS cannot be ignored in deciding how much it receives. Consequently, the ultimate amount depends somewhat on the overriding political agenda of the day. This means that although health spending is notionally about the health of the people, it is also about the political fortunes of the secretary of state for health as well as those of the government of the day.

Thus it was for New Labour in 2000 when it elevated the NHS to the very top of its political agenda. In deciding on a headline target that was intended to achieve a level of spending to match the EU average, New Labour committed itself to the NHS in an unparalleled fashion (DOH, 2000a). It did this firstly by the volume of financial increases that it offered. Secondly, the service had never previously enjoyed the promise of a long-term financial commitment of the magnitude that was proposed. It had been the convention previously to fund the NHS with only the short term in mind, and this had dogged rational forward planning for decades. What was uncertain about the sheer generosity of the proposed offer was its likely outcomes. For while it was known that the NHS showed the ability to cope with periods of financial stringency, there was no evidence of dramatic increases in its productivity and output during times of financial plenty (Appleby, 1999). This was confirmed in the early years of the new investment when this prior evidence seemed to resonate with the way that the NHS was performing.

In 2003 the Audit Commission assessed the progress of every trust in England towards meeting key *NHS Plan* targets (Audit Commission, 2003b). The Commission identified what constrained performance and what helped trusts to meet targets and the auditors also reviewed each trust's aptitude to improve its performance. The overall picture was one of good progress but evidence existed that the effects of the government's extra investment were not a universal success. Although effort had been devoted to meeting government targets, many trusts were finding it difficult to increase the numbers of frontline staff to carry out the additional work for which they were being funded. Furthermore, the majority of trusts were finding it difficult to balance the books and some had directed money intended to meet specific objectives towards more fundamental underlying financial problems. Trusts generally lacked guidelines to enable them to demonstrate and record transparently that new money had been spent to boost the services for which it was intended. Many also were unsure as to how much flexibility they had in the use of new money. The report noted that where trusts were in financial trouble, many recovery plans were unrealistic and it urged them to look beyond a lack of resources as the reason for their poor performance.

CONVINCING THE ELECTORATE: THE KEY INDICATORS OF HEALTH SPENDING

Several factors bedevil the calculation of the health care budget in arriving at what is an adequate amount. Governments in the UK have, over time, used different ways of demonstrating their financial commitment to the electorate. It can be seen from what follows that the ways in which expenditure is explained is a far from elementary matter that is open to interpretation.

TOTAL EXPENDITURE

Governments are in favour of citing the overall expenditure that they have devoted to health care. The performance of recent UK governments is illustrated in Table 4.1, which gives only a partial picture of the real expenditure on health care. For instance, it does not include government expenditure on personal social services. It also excludes the private contribution that ranges from the purchase of over-the-counter medicines to private medical insurance subscriptions. So the notion of actual health spending does, however, capture the total more accurately and takes time to calculate. Examples of this are seen in Table 4.2.

SPENDING PER HEAD OF POPULATION

Another commonly available statistic concerns the amount spent on each member of the population, or so-called 'capitation spending'. The overall mean figure per individual is available but perhaps what is a more illuminating figure is the amount spent by age group. This can be explained by the examples in Table 4.3.

Table 4.1   The total NHS budget for the years 1998/2004 (£ million)

	1998/99	1999/2000	2000/01	2001/02	2002/03	2003/04
NHS budget	Out-turn	Out-turn	Out-turn	Estimated Out-turn	Planned budget	Planned budget
	£38,794	£41,313	£44,374	£50,300	£53,948	£58,847

Source: DOH (2003g)

Table 4.2   Total (NHS plus other health spending) UK health expenditure, 1997–2001 (£ million)

	Total UK health expenditure
1997	£55,565
1998	£59,240
1999	£64,773
2000	£69,117
2001	£75,014

Source: ONS (2003)

Table 4.3   Hospital and community health expenditure: by age group of recipient, 1999–2000

Age group	£ per head of population
Birth to 4 years (includes childbirth costs)	£1,100
5 to 15 years	£198
16 to 44 years	£390
45 to 64 years	£415
65 and over	£1,390

Source: ONS (2003), adapted from Department of Health sources

What is apparent from the data in Table 4.3 is that, after relatively expensive early years, the health care of the UK population becomes less costly for most of their adult lives. It can be seen that even when the diseases of premature morbidity and mortality begin to emerge in middle age the respective population is not a financial burden. Only when people reach old age do they then become markedly more costly to the exchequer.

THE PERCENTAGE OF GROSS DOMESTIC PRODUCT AS AN INDICATOR

What has become the convention is to express the amount of government investment in terms of some notion of the overall national wealth. This has its own logic given that the funding fortunes of the NHS are tethered inevitably to what the country can afford. What can be predicted reliably is that the NHS will be treated with generosity when the overall British economy is buoyant and parsimoniously when the economy is weak. The measure used to indicate overall government concern, therefore, is frequently the percentage of gross domestic product (GDP) that is being spent on health care. Modernisation and improved investment plans for the NHS in the early 21st century was thus a consequence of low inflation and an economy that was relatively strong. The ability to fund all the future projections made by New Labour in its *NHS Plan* for modernisation and for service improvement was determined necessarily by that remaining the case.

INTERNATIONAL COMPARISONS

Having decided the percentage of GDP that the government has chosen to invest, the next temptation is to compare the figure to the amount of GDP spent by other developed countries. This mechanism is used to determine how generously a particular government is behaving towards its health services. The comparability of financial data internationally has always been problematic for several reasons. Definitions of what constitutes health care lack uniformity, statistics are collected differently from country to country and funding systems are fundamentally diverse in nature. There is the problem of erratic currency values that has eased somewhat when looking at EU comparators since the euro became more commonly embraced. Other more detailed considerations obscure the clarity of the data. For instance, the provision of care by carers and by agencies such as occupational health services in industry vary from place to place. What constitutes nursing care is also difficult to determine even within a single nation. In the UK, for instance, nursing care in England provided by a registered nurse is free. Yet that care known as 'social care' that assists with carrying out the activities of daily living that is provided by a care assistant, is means tested. In Scotland, both nursing care and social care are free. This is all further complicated by the ways in which the contributions of charities, religious organisations and non-NHS providers of health such as the prison service are treated within the data. Adding to the confusion is the way education, training and research for health is calculated in different countries.

Despite these snags, the Office of National Statistics (ONS) has in recent years been developing health accounts in the UK on an experimental basis according to an internationally agreed framework of concepts, definitions, classifications and accounting rules, drawn up by the Organisation for Economic Co-operation and Development (OECD) that represents the world's richest nations (ONS, 2003).

Table 4.4   Total expenditure as a percentage of GDP: international comparisons, 1997–2001

	1997	1998	1999	2000	2001
Australia	8.5	8.6	8.7	8.9	
Austria	8.0	8.0	8.0	8.0	
Belgium	8.5	8.5	8.7	8.7	
Canada	8.9	9.1	9.1	9.2	9.7
Czech Republic	7.1	7.1	7.1	7.1	7.3
Denmark	8.2	8.4	8.5	8.3	8.6
Finland	7.3	6.9	6.9	6.7	7.0
France	9.4	9.3	9.3	9.3	9.5
Germany	10.7	10.6	10.6	10.6	10.7
Greece	9.4	9.4	9.6	9.4	9.4
Hungary	7.0	6.9	6.8	6.7	6.8
Iceland	8.1	8.5	8.9	9.1	
Ireland	6.4	6.2	6.2	6.4	6.5
Italy	7.7	7.7	7.8	8.2	8.4
Japan	6.8	7.1	7.5	7.6	
Korea	5.0	5.1	5.6	5.9	
Luxembourg	5.9	5.8	6.1	5.6	
Mexico	5.4	5.2	5.5	5.6	6.6
Netherlands	8.2	8.6	8.7	8.6	8.9
New Zealand	7.5	8.0	7.9	8.0	8.2
Norway	7.8	8.5	8.5	7.7	8.3
Poland	6.1	6.4	6.2		
Portugal	8.6	8.6	8.7	9.0	9.2
Spain	7.5	7.5	7.5	7.5	7.5
Sweden	8.2	8.3	8.4	8.4	8.7
Switzerland	10.4	10.6	10.7	10.7	10.9
Turkey	4.2	4.8			
UK	6.8	6.9	7.2	7.3	7.6
USA	13.0	13.0	13.0	13.1	13.9

Source: OECD (2003)

Health accounts provide a comprehensive, coherent, standardised and consistent statistical description of health care expenditure. As such, they provide meaningful comparisons over time as well as across countries. Many countries in the European Union as well as the OECD group of countries and more globally are taking steps to develop publicly available health accounts; publicly available estimates for other countries can be found on the OECD website (www.oecd.org). International comparisons on the percentage of GDP spent on health care are shown in Table 4.4.

Despite the contentious nature of the notion of GDP as an indicator of health spending and notwithstanding the debate about the validity of international comparisons, New Labour chose to use this indicator. In 2000, in

Table 4.5 Experimental total UK health expenditure estimates, 1997–2001 (£ million)

	Total health expenditure (£m)	As a percentage of GDP
1997	£55,565	6.8
1998	£59,240	6.9
1999	£64,773	7.2
2000	£69,117	7.3
2001	£75,014	7.6

Source: ONS (2003)

a remark made initially in a television interview, Tony Blair committed the government to achieving the average spending on health of other European Union countries of 8 per cent of GDP by 2006 and exceeding it by 2008 (BBC, 2000).

The New Labour commitment to the European figure of 8 per cent of GDP by 2006 presupposed that health spending across the then 15 nations would remain stable and, furthermore, that it was a rational target at which to aim. It has been argued, however, that the EU mean for health spending had been underestimated by as much as 1 per cent and that the volume of compensatory spending that would be needed by the UK to achieve it, would be correspondingly deficient (Towse and Sussex, 2000; Emmerson et al., 2002). Examples of the estimates of the percentage of GDP that have been spent on health in Britain can be seen in Table 4.5.

Choosing the EU mean assumes that the UK investment in health care has been lower than might have been expected. Yet it can be argued that the UK system is considerably more efficient administratively than health systems elsewhere in Europe and worldwide. Revenue is collected mainly from general taxation through compulsory 'pay as you earn' (PAYE) deductions from wages and salaries at source. This is a managerially convenient mechanism for raising and distributing resources. Health care that is largely free at the point it is received also avoids cumbersome procedures for settling bills for treatment and this adds to its economic efficiency. The central planning of major facilities also attempts to secure sufficient NHS bed capacity but to avoid wasteful spare capacity that adds to its good organisation. The use of salaried doctors and other salaried professionals is less wasteful than in European systems where patients are charged a fee for every item of service they receive. This encourages over-investigation and over-treatment that inflates costs that are then added to by further lengthy accounting and invoicing procedures that increase the overheads for treatment. Consideration of these factors suggests that the NHS has much to commend it in terms of its economic prudence when compared, for example, with the USA. The USA spends almost twice as much as a percentage of its GDP as Britain on its health care but still has an estimated 41 million residents that lack any form of health insurance (Marwick, 2003). The uninsured have poorer health, live shorter lives, receive inadequate health care and frequently receive it so late that it costs the individuals and the state many billions of dollars. Against this evidence, therefore, it seems reasonable to claim that the NHS produces a very respectable volume and quality of care for a seemingly modest financial outlay.

RAISING THE REVENUE

The need to properly fund health care catches the public imagination and is founded on the misunderstanding that modern medicine can almost always do something useful. Politicians reinforce the case that better health services and a better NHS means better health. The demand for its services is thus unstoppable. Yet in terms of the improved distribution of the available funds, there is a reasoned case that spending on clinical interventions is only a partial solution, given that the origins of ill health are also socio-economic and behavioural. The corollary is that the government should be spending more on health promotion, disease prevention, housing and social services.

Governments strive continuously to make better use of existing investment. This begins by attempting to optimise resource allocation so that money is spent where it achieves the maximum return for the initial outlay. Efficiency savings and improved productivity are also at the heart of policy with providers being charged to deliver more care in a year from the same amount of investment that was made in the previous year. On this basis, the more efficient they become, the more difficult it becomes to get even more efficient in the future. The enhancement of clinical effectiveness by employing treatment protocols that convey best value for money is a similar priority as is improved prescribing efficiency. Yet despite a relentless approach to effectiveness and efficiency, the question about how to best raise more resources recurs.

Funding is inevitably at the root of any debate about the NHS and all of the structural reorganisations of it are predicated on the belief that these will improve its economic efficiency. In generating the necessary resources and improving the economic performance of the NHS, governments have several principal alternatives that can be defined as follows:

- general taxation;
- hypothecated taxes;
- social insurance;

- private medical insurance;
- patient charges;
- public–private partnerships and the private finance initiative.

GENERAL TAXATION

General taxation has provided the major funding stream for the NHS and seems likely to do so not least of all because the outcomes of a change to any alternative source is untested and would be difficult to forecast. As a funding supply it has much to commend it because it is cheap to collect. It draws from a broad constituency mainly of those in employment whose contribution is proportionate to their earnings and who arguably can afford to pay the tax, so this makes it a fair method. It is also sufficiently adaptable in that its rate can be altered according to national needs.

Yet as the principal source of revenue general taxation is politically potent and this determines the feasibility of manipulating its use at any particular time. Chancellors of the exchequer have the option to divert money from other items of public expenditure to the NHS such as education, road building or defence, but this runs the risk of political unpopularity through depriving those services of resources. Similarly, there is a hazard for any government considering an increase in income tax, and a commitment not to do this is a feature of many pre-election manifestos. New Labour committed itself not to increase the rate of general taxation in both of its first two terms in office but threatened in its second term that this might be necessary to finance its ambitious *NHS Plan*.

New Labour committed itself in the long term to an NHS that was to be funded by general taxation in its unequivocal acceptance of a report that visualised how a high quality health service might be provided into the future (HM Treasury, 2002a). A former chief executive of the National Westminster Bank, Derek Wanless, was commissioned to estimate projections of resources required over the subsequent 20 years by considering a range of possibilities for the future through three alternative resourcing models. The resulting projections showed that the UK would need to be spending between 10.6 and 12.5 per cent of GDP on health care by 2022–23, compared to 7.7 per cent in 2002. The average annual real terms growth rate required for UK NHS spending was estimated to be between 4.2 and 5.1 per cent per annum over the 20-year period.

These forecasts were defined in five-year blocks that showed that the highest growth in spending in the early part of the review period with an average of between 7.1 and 7.3 per cent per annum in real terms needed over the first five years. This level of spending was claimed by the report to reflect the need for significant investment to allow the NHS to 'catch up' to perceived standards internationally and to create the ability to expand user choice in future. The report stressed that the pace of growth must be considered within the context of the service's capacity. It noted also that its predictions were at the upper end of what should be sensibly spent.

The Wanless proposals linked distinct service developments to the cash that would be required to pay for them that included:

- An increase in health spending from £68 billion in 2002 to £184 billion by 2022.
- Proportion of GDP spent on health to rise from 7.7 per cent in 2002 to 12.5 per cent by 2022.
- NHS spending to increase by 7.7 per cent from 2002 for the next five years, reaching £96 billion by 2007.
- A one-third increase in the number of nurses.
- A two-thirds increase in the number of doctors.
- A maximum two-week waiting time for hospital appointments by 2022.
- Improvements to NHS pay and new financial incentives to encourage staff to improve services.
- NHS staff must increase productivity from 2 per cent a year at present to 2.5 per cent a year in the first 10 years if improvements are to be made.
- A doubling of spending on information technology was required.
- A major increase in the new hospitals building programme to bring the average age of facilities down to 30 years.
- Redistribution of tasks between NHS staff: health assistants taking over some of the work of nurses and nurses taking over some of the responsibilities of doctors.
- A study to be conducted to consider whether patients should be charged for missing NHS appointments.
- Greater patient involvement in the running of the NHS and related organisations such as the National Institute for Clinical Excellence.
- A review of the policy that exempts up to 50 per cent of the population from paying prescription charges.
- The introduction of charges for non-clinical services such as food and laundry.
- Greater co-operation between the NHS and the private sector.
- Financial incentives to reduce delayed discharges from NHS hospitals.
- More self-care by patients.

- If successful, the NHS will help to increase life expectancy for men from 80 years at present to 81.6 years, and for women from 83.8 years to 85.5 years by 2002.
- Greater integration between the NHS and social services.
- A review of the progress being made in improving the NHS and a re-assessment of its future needs in 2007.

The Conservative Party rejected this as a solution to the long-term improvement of care and predicted that higher rates of income tax would result from the Wanless proposals. The utopian nature of the proposals was also a common concern and the vastness of their scope and their feasibility was questioned (Moore, 2002). The final version of the report aroused the same criticisms that had accompanied its interim version four months earlier (HM Treasury, 2001). These had questioned the dependence of the plan on Britain avoiding economic recession (Klein, 2001). The use of the EU average was also disputed on the grounds of the reliability of its meaning and its relevance as a benchmark to British circumstances. Wanless supported patient choice but there was no clarity about the cost consequences for this. The alternatives to general taxation as a method of funding health care were all rejected. Private care was discarded and it was suggested that this and social insurance models are more costly, inequitable and still do not confer patients the degree of choice that has been assumed for them. Almost every UK government since the inception of the NHS has considered alternatives to general taxation to fund the NHS. Wanless therefore was not atypical in reaching the decision similar to others before him who have also concluded that a tax-funded system does not depend on the ability to pay, is the cheapest to administer and is the most equitable because of its intentions to redistribute from those with means to those without.

HYPOTHECATED OR EARMARKED HEALTH TAXES

The national insurance (NI) stamp was intended in 1948 to serve partly as an earmarked tax for the NHS but there was no appreciation at the time of the demands that would eventually be made on it by the benefits system. In the Budget of April 2003, the Chancellor added an increase in NI of 1 per cent for all workers earning more than £4,615, which had the same effect as a 1p rise in income tax rates across the board. It was estimated at the time that a worker with the average UK salary of £21,400 would pay an extra £3.70 a week.

Further up the income scale, a worker earning £50,000 a year became £453.85 a year worse off, while a counterpart bringing in £100,000 a year had to pay an extra £953.85 a year. This comprised a big political gamble and provided a semi-plausible yet inaccurate observation that the New Labour government had not really increased general taxation. The Chancellor used the rise in NI to pay for the UK's biggest ever increase in health service funding. The increase on both employer's and employee's contributions funded a £40 billion growth in NHS spending over five years. This provoked a more enduring argument about the introduction of an earmarked health tax. While the public might be willing to pay more towards a fund that is dedicated to health care, it is less certain whether they would be willing to pay more tax. The protagonists for a ring-fenced fund would argue that the NHS should have a dedicated resource that is outside the control of government to protect it from the financial fluctuations that hindered its development during its history. While New Labour had committed itself in the long term to such an arrangement, its promises could become unsustainable if economic recession were to occur.

The advantages of a health tax are that it could be raised independently of the normal political process and might make health care a less controversial issue politically. Yet the overall proposal is unlikely to find favour with MPs who would not wish to relinquish control by the Treasury of such a vast item of public expenditure. Furthermore, an independent agency to manage the fund would be required and this could be prohibitively costly to operate. Having a more transparent fund than exists currently could also leave government a hostage to fortune concerning the extent of the demands that certain sectors of the NHS workforce might make.

To raise the revenue to sustain a high quality service that caters fairly for all its users would require a compulsory health tax. This raises questions about whether it would really be different from the present system of general taxation through the collection of income tax. Furthermore, a health tax would be raised principally to support treatment and caring services and this could be a distraction from and a disadvantage to tackling the socio-economic causes of ill health arising from deprivation, poor housing and unemployment.

SOCIAL INSURANCE

Under social insurance schemes that are employed in Europe, individuals and employees donate through a payroll tax and the state contributes for the unemployed by drawing from general taxation. Those with dependants either insure them separately or are assisted to do so by the state. In the

UK the most feasible way of raising social insurance would be through the NI contribution and this would presumably need to be assisted by a corresponding reduction in income tax. Contributions in European social insurance schemes can be at different levels of cover and quality and can require different additional personal payments when services are accessed. Contributions go to a sickness fund or competing sickness funds that are run on a 'not-for-profit' basis. Fund managers bargain with providers for the most favourable packages of care and pay for this on the subscribers' behalf. Social insurance would have to be compulsory to work effectively and therefore it does not differ sufficiently from either general or hypothecated taxation to justify its implementation. Wanless rejected social insurance on the basis that it is more costly to administer than general taxation and believed that it sacrifices equity for groups that are more vulnerable economically (HM Treasury, 2002a).

PRIVATE MEDICAL INSURANCE

Private insurance has historically made little financial contribution to the NHS because its benefits were largely spent on treatments in the private hospital sector. But the NHS is now the largest provider of private elective surgery that accounts for most of the activity conducted for the privately insured. Managers have realised that competition with private hospitals for elective work is worthwhile because it provides a funding stream in addition to that from the exchequer and earnings from private patients have become a substantial source of income generation. There is even perhaps scope for more of this activity through concessionary deals for private patients that might be struck with the insurance industry. The Independent Health Care Association has, however, called for private work in the NHS to be curtailed and has questioned the fairness of competition with it (IHA, 2002).

The Conservatives are the only party with an explicit policy to encourage private medical insurance and its uptake rose during their period in office from 2 per cent of the population in 1979 to 13 per cent in 1997, a figure that has remained relatively stable. The Conservative Party, along with its other champions on the political right, argue that parts of the NHS could be funded privately because certain services are luxuries and should be insured against to meet the full cost, or that the state should only bear the burden of a portion of treatment costs and this should be topped up by the patient. It is thus believed that encouraging or compelling more people to insure to supplement their treatment costs would reduce the overall level of taxation as more individuals became less dependent on state-funded services. Certainly tax inducements to individuals could provide an incentive to take out a medical insurance policy that is the necessary precursor to enlarging the private health sector that the Conservative Party would wish for. The party has claimed that those who pay for care and treatment either through a policy or from individual payments are to be congratulated for exercising personal choice and also for taking pressure off the NHS (Fox, 2002).

The idea of replenishing NHS provision through the use of private medical insurance raises the thought that it might become a 'core' service. This presumes that the state will perhaps always wish to take responsibility for life-threatening illnesses. But it might elect to restrict the universalist principles on which the NHS was founded by defining a 'core' of restricted services that it opts to provide with patients purchasing private medical insurance for those things outside the 'core', or making individual out-of-pocket payments for them. The drawback within this option concerns which services might comprise the core and how these should be defined in terms of both ethical and economic rationality. While the similar experience in the famous Oregon experiment led to failure to define the 'core', there is nevertheless sufficient evidence that the core service concept is alive, even if in embryonic form, given that the NHS has virtually precluded its purchase of some procedures such as IVF, tattoo removal and the reversal of sterilisation operations (Bodenheimer, 1997a, 1997b). What is required is not so much a definition of what exclusions should exist but more a priority setting mechanism that identifies the cost benefits to those individuals who will be treated. The inherent problem with the core service idea is the determination of where both state and private market responsibilities were to begin and end.

With any form of extended model of private medical insurance a large number of the population would not be insurable and insurance companies that exist for profit, would aim to attract the least risky subscribers. They also would have exclusions for the most expensive treatments and packages of care. In addition, those without means to sustain insurance premiums would require some state provision to meet their needs. Advocates for the more wholesale introduction of private medical insurance argue that it:

- Is founded on the premise of consumer sovereignty where the paying customers seek the best deal and would be free to take their custom elsewhere.
- Reduces demand for public funding and results in less personal taxation.
- Brings in a mobile, private financial resource that results in more consumer-responsive providers. This stimulates innovation, more personally tailored care and results in a reduction in waiting times.

- Produces more cost-conscious users because by knowing the true economic cost of an episode of treatment, insurance subscribers would be careful not to overuse services that might increase their premium. Additionally, economic awareness would lead to more self-care and more health awareness.
- Behaves as a safety valve for the NHS by relieving it of elective cases.

Against these main supporting arguments for private medical insurance its opponents claim that it:

- Relies on market competition and produces higher transaction costs than a state-controlled system that has lower overheads.
- Is parasitic on the NHS for its personnel because it does little in the way of pre-registration training of the major health professions.
- It similarly scrounges on the NHS and is subsidised by the state through its heavy reliance on the spare capacity of NHS consultants. The reliance on NHS consultants means that, technologically, its benefits are no greater than the NHS, although its customer and hotel services convey greater overall convenience.
- Personifies the existence of a social class divide because it is based on the ability to pay that gives subscribers the right-to-buy priority. It thus discriminates against the poorest in the population who are made to wait for treatment.
- Forfeits comprehensiveness because insurance companies have prohibited categories of ill health for conditions such as mental illness and chronic degenerative diseases.
- Is unlikely that private insurance companies can be interested in public health and population health prevention strategies.
- Has the potential to relegate the NHS to a sub-standard service for the least fortunate in society.

The extent to which the introduction of private health insurance into British health care would be judged in terms of its feasibility has several interacting determinants. The predominant consideration is political and concerns its impact on access that becomes immediately based on personal financial means and the ability to pay rather than on access that is dictated by clinical need. This makes even the political right suspect whether it is practicable. Even with the most ambitious move to privatise the NHS, the extent of state provision that would have to remain as a safety net for the uninsurable and the poor might become a good reason for not proceeding. With an increasingly ageing population that would probably mean that a large state presence would be necessary. There is a further assumption that what remained of the NHS would provide good quality services if it were not to become third rate. This leads to a further proviso: a still substantial, good quality NHS would have to be funded by the taxpayer and it is by no means certain that those who are insured privately would be ready and willing to contribute for a second time for a service they never intend to use.

PATIENT CHARGES

A significant feature of the NHS in relation to its international comparators is the very low level of patient charges that it expects. This therefore is clearly an area worthy of exploration in attempting to increase the availability of resources. Two considerations are worthwhile in the initial reflection on this option. The first is at a theoretical level in that supporters of more charges argue that paying for services confers personal choice and the expression of a preference that is not generally available when accessing state services. Against this is the political imagery that charging invokes as a device for undermining the motives of the welfare state. What is certain is that patient charges discourage the uptake of services. This is well illustrated by the introduction of an almost privately run optician service in the UK that severely curtailed the uptake of eye tests. A similar reduction of uptake resulted from an increasingly privatised dental service. Patient charges also establish the provision of services on the ability to pay rather than on clinical need and require an accompanying exemptions policy for the poor who might go without treatment. Therein lies a second major issue in relation to the level at which to set any particular charge. If the charge is set too low it may be uneconomical to collect. If the charge is set too high it might be similarly self-defeating if too many people are exempt, making it not worthwhile to collect.

A further question arises: which charges should be obligatory and which should be voluntary? Patient charges for prescriptions exist compulsorily for certain members of the population but have a high exemption rate. Charges may also be paid voluntarily for ophthalmic and dental services. This is complicated by the need for intricate and bureaucratic financial systems to manage and to both properly make payments to practitioners who provide services and also to guard against fraudulent claims being made by them.

Discussion from time to time has suggested that the introduction of a broader range of individual payments is necessary. Examples considered have included charges for GP night visits, GP home visits, GP surgery consultations, hospital transportation and hotel services for in-patient treatment. Extending patient charges could induce a further privatisation and act as an inspiration to insure against those things that patients might otherwise have to pay for out of their pocket.

In reality, charging has become unwieldy both politically and practically. The adverse effect on access and anomalies in exemption rules is a disincentive to widen the scope of patient charges. Furthermore, in relation to general taxation, patient charges are correspondingly less efficient because all of those who are not exempt pay at the same rate irrespective of the size of their income.

PUBLIC–PRIVATE PARTNERSHIPS AND PRIVATE FINANCE

Borrowing money from the private sector is another prominent means of raising finances to support the NHS. NHS trust hospitals were first given powers to raise private capital in 1991 but Treasury rules had strictly curtailed the amounts they could borrow. Relaxation of the borrowing rules came with public–private partnerships (PPPs), the first of which concerned the private finance initiative (PFI). The Conservative government introduced the PFI in the mid-1990s as a series of one-off schemes. Labour at the time was vehemently opposed to what it saw as further demolition of the welfare state and had vowed to abolish these schemes. But by the time it assumed office in 1997, it embraced the PFI with a vigorous affection that was unsurpassed by its predecessors.

New Labour's attachment to thinking that was in continuity with Thatcherism was to see a shift in the intended equilibrium of health care delivery in the UK between the state and the non-state sectors (Butler and Yarrow, 2001). The key difference between PFI and conventional ways of providing public services is that the public and the state do not own the asset. The NHS makes an annual payment to the private company that provides the building and associated services, rather like a mortgage. A company is set up especially to run the scheme and will typically own a PFI project. These companies usually operate as consortiums comprising a building firm, a bank and a facilities management company. Whilst PFI projects can be structured in different ways, there are usually four key elements: design, finance, build and operate.

The first thorough dispassionate evaluation of PPPs resulted from the Commission on Public–Private Partnerships that reported in 2001 (IPPR, 2001). The Commissioners comprised leading thinkers, ranging from public and private sector managers, academics and trade unionists, that initiated a new direction for the public services in the UK. Following extensive consultation across public, private and voluntary sectors, the

Commission introduced a new lucidity to PPPs and produced a convincing protocol to inform the use of these in the future. This made radical proposals on where, when and how PPPs had a role and how this might be expanded to enhance the delivery of public services. The report quickly impacted on approaches to NHS reform, and its immediate effect was for government to use it to urge the NHS to consider private solutions to what previously had been regarded as public service problems.

What the report believed had been easily underestimated was the potential opportunities that could be created through a mixed economy in health care services. This enables the state to convert the users of services into consumers by offering them choice. By doing so, competition is stimulated between providers in the interests of achieving better value for money for the taxpayer. This need not necessarily reduce state control and there is the capacity to increase state leverage through stronger regulatory powers that improve both the volume and quality of available services.

The original PFI schemes used private capital to build new hospitals and were followed by NHS local improvement finance trusts (LIFT) for the development of primary health care facilities. These paved the way for more enduring PPPs. New Labour instigated more ambitious developments in its second term as it moved towards a greater plurality of services. This included plans to:

- use the under-occupancy of private hospital beds to treat NHS patients requiring elective surgery under a concordat with the acute private hospital providers;
- introduce NHS-purchased intermediate care for elderly people in the privately run nursing home and rest home sector;
- create independent not-for-profit foundation hospitals;
- recruit private companies from abroad to increase NHS capacity in the provision of diagnostic and elective surgical services (DOH, 2002b).

New Labour's second-term manifesto maxim for health care concerned the use of 'what works best' (Labour Party, 2001). Yet it had no clear rationale for PPPs or evidence that long-term contracts with private providers work in the public interest. In fact, the issue of transparency concerning value for money from PPP and PFI schemes was questioned seriously by the government's own Health Select Committee (Stationery Office, 2002).

The Comptroller and Auditor General identified that PPPs and PFIs had introduced considerable changes in the way that public services were to be procured (Stationery Office, 2001b). PPP and PFI contracts identify performance levels and specify financial sanctions that will be levied if the agreed performance is not achieved. But there are key issues of which public authorities must be mindful when managing relationships with private contractors. Within successful partnerships the focus was noted to be on working together and securing mutual benefits. This mutual success was characterised by value for money for the public sector and a reasonable return for the contractor.

Public authorities engaging in PFI and PPPs had high expectations of contractors. But careful monitoring and project management was required and public authorities needed to consult with their service users on their level of satisfaction with what was being provided. Contractors often commence with a different set of objectives from their public sector counterparts. To be successful the venture has to be approached in a spirit of co-operation. Participants have to understand each other's business and develop a common vision. Where this had not occurred, adversarial relationships were found (Stationery Office, 2001b). Parameters for a successful partnership need to be set early and included within the contract to allocate risk appropriately and establish clearly defined quality and performance criteria that become necessary as the project evolves. Having staff with the right skills and training is crucial to contract management. A good partnership is one where both sides share information and work together to solve problems. Both public authorities and contractors need to review their relationships and monitoring arrangements on a regular basis to see how improved governance can maintain them.

THE OPPOSITION TO PRIVATE SECTOR INVOLVEMENT

The trade unions have an ideological objection to private finance in all its forms (IPPR, 2002). They believe that the private sector should have no part in public services but in fact organisations such as private building companies have always been involved in building hospitals. The trade unions also allege that these schemes are a form of back-door privatisation.

The fundamental interest of private health care providers is profit and they are naturally selective about those services that will yield a profit. Equally they are keen to leave financially unattractive tasks for the NHS to deal with by itself. Additionally, private providers are vulnerable to distorting priorities and to cutting corners that sacrifice efficiency and quality in order to increase their profit margins. The mixed economy in health service provision has therefore been criticised on the grounds that it has failed to ask more fundamental questions about the role of markets and for-profit operators (Pollock et al., 2001, Stationery Office, 2002). This view holds that the claim that competition delivers value for money is unfounded and underplays the limitations of the cost and efficiency of PPPs and PFI that are not only earmarking increasing amounts of public money, but also give a guaranteed income to private profit-making corporations for decades to come. In the case of the NHS, for example, the PFI is seemingly reducing the number of beds that are available for use. It remedies its lack of capacity and simultaneously subsidises the private sector by contracting out the work with which it cannot cope. It is argued thereby that there is neither an economic nor a morally defensible case for forcing the NHS to direct taxpayers' money towards private providers (Pollock et al., 2001, 2002).

International evidence and that from the UK social care sector is cited to confirm that private sector involvement confers no consistent benefits in either cost quality or efficiency (Pollock et al., 2001). It is further supposed that private providers are potentially unaccountable and that PFIs and PPPs can trap the NHS into a contract in ways that make it tolerate poor performance. In consequence, the NHS runs the risk of forgoing its legal and regulatory rights simply because it has no alternative supplier. Opponents maintain that nowhere in the world has a universal, equitable health service of the type unique to Britain been delivered where a salient profit-making element exists.

From this perspective, therefore, the key to reforming the NHS is not the profit motive but democracy and accountability.

CONCLUSION

The solutions to the infinite demands made upon the NHS are complex and have always been seen in terms of raising more public finance. With the inexorable growth in health care, questions necessarily arise about the longer-term appropriateness of a nationalised, publicly funded health care system that has its origins in the 1940s. The fact that the UK has spent less historically than most industrialised countries on its health care does not provide a prima facie case for spending more. New Labour's ambitious policies provided compensatory funding for the NHS. It inherited a service in 1997 that consumed 6.8 per cent of GDP, and within its first term committed itself to spend the EU weighted average of 8 per cent of GDP by 2006. It similarly pledged to continue to fund the NHS largely from general taxation, thus rejecting the need for more funding from the alternative sources that have been considered in this chapter.

Although all governments consider funding the NHS by means that are alternative to general taxation, they are all left with an identical dilemma. Funding by any other method would inevitably be either more costly and less efficient or it would threaten the founding principles on which the service was conceived and created. Social insurance is an example of this where, in France and Germany, it is not only expensive to administer but it also requires user payments to enable it to work fully (HM Treasury, 2002a). Likewise, more widespread use of private medical insurance would threaten equal access on the basis of need, undermine comprehensiveness and, if enough of the population opted for it, could undermine the public commitment to the NHS, thereby running the risk of it becoming sub-standard. Patient charges would be similarly detrimental to access if an adequate exemptions system were not in place and this too would incur high transaction costs in its administration that would inevitably be more complicated than what exists presently.

Perhaps the most radical palpable departure from the conventional approach to raising money for the NHS resides within the debate about the various merits of either public spending or the use of private capital. Superficially, private capital provides new money that seems cheap at the outset because it does not require the Treasury to make an initial outlay in the way that publicly funded projects used to be managed. Furthermore, privately financed projects do not appear in the public sector borrowing requirement figures so they do not look like a public liability. Yet in the longer term, critics of private finance point to the true extent of the debt that has to be serviced through the payment of interest over many years. The reality is that the taxpayer ultimately funds private finance and there is little convincing evidence either way of its value for money (IPPR, 2002). What is also certain is that the taxpayer is also liable to pick up the costs of any privately financed project that fails.

Ultimately the NHS is left with the same conclusion. This concerns getting the maximum return from what it spends. It has historically worked on a ritualistic basis that did things in particular ways without questioning why. All the scientific evidence points to the need for improved measurement of costs and benefits. This endeavour will doubtless continue because the risk of tinkering with the fundamental taxation-funded arrangements is too mighty to contemplate. It has nevertheless to be acknowledged that the challenge to those spending for better health services is overwhelmingly complicated and there is no ready-made mechanism for fixing priorities. Yet political expediency will inevitably be the determinant of government spending decisions because in the final analysis it is ministers who carry the blame if service delivery falls short of public expectations.

FIVE

WHO CONTROLS THE NHS?

INTRODUCTION

The NHS is an esteemed institution despite any critics it may have and this, as has been illustrated repeatedly in previous chapters, adds to its intense politicisation. This chapter will analyse the organisation, direction and control of the service that have proven so difficult to secure throughout its history. The chapter will selectively consider the relative contribution of the major aspects of power and control that will include:

- The macro-management of the NHS: its regulation.
- The micro-management of the NHS: its organisational context.
- Medical power.
- Doctors and managers in the modernised NHS.

Ultimately the secretary of state for health is in charge of the NHS. Through the Civil Service and the Department of Health and its subordinate agencies, government policy is intended to be cascaded in a linear fashion through the various levels of the service and translated into practical action wherever patients are treated. A feature of New Labour, however, has been the influence on policy that is exerted by sources outside the Civil Service by academic theorists, special advisers and, by no means least, the party's media managers (Hunter, 2002). Policy can also be a knee-jerk response to critical or adverse events as will be seen later in the chapter.

THE MACRO-MANAGEMENT OF THE NHS: ITS REGULATION

A startling feature of the modernised NHS that has accompanied its intensive central political control by government, has been the piecemeal emergence of a number of regulatory bodies, the range and scope of which leave even diligent students of the service perplexed. These bodies act variously towards NHS trusts as inspectorial, advisory, or a mixture of the two. The regulatory bodies have been created, on the one hand, to be quasi-independent of government yet, on the other, to steer the service in the direction that government policy makers have set for it. These bodies will be considered as follows.

THE MODERNISATION AGENCY

The NHS Modernisation Agency was established in April 2001 to provide strategic support in initiating the *NHS Plan* and improving leadership (DOH, 2000a). It discharges its function alongside strategic health authorities, primary care trusts and NHS trusts to implement local delivery plans (LDPs). The Agency embraces a breadth of expertise including the following:

- Leadership Centre;
- National Primary and Care Trust Development Programme (NatPaCT);
- National Primary Care Development Team;
- NHS Clinical Governance Support Team;
- Service Improvement Team.

The major focus of its endeavour concerns:

- Quicker access to a GP.
- Leadership skills training of over 40,000 NHS staff.
- Supporting all zero-star trusts through a programme of co-ordinated action.
- Co-ordinating the continued growth in the numbers of all booked appointments at a date and time of the patient's choice.
- Co-ordinating collaboration of cancer care services.
- Co-ordinating the development of Critical Care Networks.

By 2004 the staff of the Modernisation Agency had grown to 760 and government decided that from April 2005 this would be reduced to 150 in a new successor organisation (DOH, 2004a). The existing functions were to be transferred with the necessary staff to a much more local level.

THE COMMISSION FOR HEALTH IMPROVEMENT (CHI)

CHI was the first NHS inspectorate to be set up in 2000. It was independent of the NHS. Its reports were available on the public records and it highlighted where the NHS was working well and it identified the areas that needed improvement. It aimed therefore to reduce unacceptable variations in care and to ensure that every NHS patient received the highest level of service. The patient's experience was at the heart of CHI's work. Its remit included:

- Monitoring clinical governance systems in NHS trusts.
- Investigating serious service failures.
- Reporting on key issues such as coronary heart disease.
- Publishing performance data including the performance ratings.
- Publishing data on staff and patient surveys.
- Conducting joint inspections with other bodies.
- Managing the clinical audit programme.
- Ensuring the recommendations of the National Institute for Clinical Excellence (NICE) were implemented.
- Assessing performance against targets set within National Service Frameworks (NSFs).
- Identifying where improvement was required and sharing good practice within the service, thus helping the NHS to raise standards of patient care.

The CHI was created initially to conduct clinical governance reviews that formed a significant portion of its work. Review teams were multi-professional and comprised an NHS doctor, nurse, a professional allied to medicine, a lay member and an NHS manager. These reviewers were supplemented to reflect the nature of the organisation under review. A CHI review manager led and managed the team for the duration of the review exercise.

The notion of clinical governance stemmed from a consultation on quality in the new NHS that originated from the NHS Executive (NHS Executive, 1998). Its principal tenets are to:

- Introduce national consistency in the introduction of evidence-based practice including the adoption of guidelines emerging from the assessments made by NICE.
- Improve quality control and assurance.
- Improve local professional regulation and deal with poor performance.
- Improve accountability and transparency.

NICE was initiated as a Special Health Authority for England and Wales in April 1999. It is part of the NHS role to disseminate information about *best practice* to patients, health professionals and the public. Its intention is to provide the NHS with authoritative, robust and reliable advice and on current individual health technologies. These embrace new medicines, medical devices, diagnostic techniques and procedure, as well as the clinical management of specific conditions. It is the adoption of this evidence that CHI was to ensure happened in trusts and PCTs that it inspected.

It has always been assumed tacitly that clinical care achieved parity of standards for individual interventions across the entire NHS. This was called into question in early pronouncements from the first New Labour government (DOH, 1997). This was reinforced by subsequent policy that prescribed a new ambitious strategy for quality enhancement (DOH 1998a, 2000a).

The objectives of NSFs are to:

- set national standards and identify key interventions for a defined service or care group;
- put in place strategies to support implementation;
- establish ways to ensure progress within an agreed timescale;
- form one of a range of measures to raise quality and decrease variations in service and to act as key drivers in delivering the modernisation agenda.

There is usually only one new framework a year and each NSF is developed with the assistance of an External Reference Group (ERG) which brings together health professionals, service users and carers, health service managers, partner agencies, and other advocates. ERGs adopt an inclusive process to engage the full range of views. The Department of Health supports the ERGs and manages the overall process of NSF development.

The rolling programme of NSFs was launched in April 1998 and covers:

- frameworks on cancer that were established at the time;
- paediatric intensive care;
- diabetes;
- mental health;
- coronary heart disease;
- national cancer plan;
- older people;
- renal services;
- children's services;
- long-term conditions focusing on neurological conditions;
- agreement with the Association of the British Pharmaceutical Agency.

This clearly represents a very broad-ranging agenda for action and it has been the remit of CHI to assess the individual progress of trusts and PCTs against these standards. Furthermore, given the concentration of New Labour on improving access to elective care, this departure represents recognition of chronic and intractable diseases that provide a major logistical and financial challenge to the NHS (Lewis and Dixon, 2004).

The CHI's brief rapidly expanded to oversee other inspectorates, and although it commenced gently it came under ministerial pressure to become more judgemental and it did so (Day and Kline, 2002). As it began to be evaluated during its early operation, the biggest criticism of it was the inconsistency in its reporting (NHS Confederation, 2003). In reviewing its reports it was observed that no two were the same and that there was a strong focus on non-clinical issues such as car parking and patients' views about hospital catering (Day and Kline, 2002).

The NHS Confederation, an organisation that represents NHS trusts, in a representative sample survey of its member organisations, noted that a quarter of trusts found the inspection process to be an unhelpful experience (NHS Confederation, 2003). Those claiming this cited their main concerns with the review process. These were the appropriateness of the inspection methodology to the actual organisation, its impartiality and robustness, its tone and style, and its lack of uniformity. Dissatisfied organisations felt that the CHI had not taken the actual evolution of their organisational milieu into account, especially where trust mergers and reorganisation had recently occurred and where the magnitude of change that staff had under-gone had been ignored. Complainants felt the review process had been inquisitorial rather than developmental and there had been a lack of clarity about data the trust had been asked to collect and poor communication about how it was actually to be used by the reviewers.

The CHI was also charged as another contentious function to manage the performance rating methodology, known colloquially as the 'star rating' system. This uses a complex formulaic data-collection exercise. The data are made up of information about delivery targets that match the government's policy agenda such as waiting times and financial targets, plus targets concerning clinical performance, patient satisfaction and staff opinions. The respective data are treated variously but are aggregated eventually into a single score that is meant to summarise the quality of performance of local trusts and PCTs. This score is intended to inform the general public to help them to better understand how their local NHS providers are performing. Essentially, star ratings are meant to smooth out variations in performance of NHS trusts and PCTs and increase their local accountability. For trust hospitals, performance indicators have been a norm for over a decade but for PCTs that have been relatively unpoliced this represented a considerable challenge.

The aggregate performance score is converted to a number of stars that are linked to managerial autonomy so that three-star trusts are eligible for full autonomy as foundation hospitals. Two-star trusts have some autonomy but require help from the Modernisation Agency and are man-aged lightly by their strategic health authority. One-star trusts also need more substantial support of the Modernisation Agency and are perfor-mance managed more rigorously by their strategic health authority. Zero-star trusts have three months to prepare a recovery plan and are supported by the Modernisation Agency. These alleged worst performers may be considered for franchising to another more successful NHS trust or to a private management company if they are not seen able to rectify their deficiencies.

The problem with this performance rating exercise concerns the arbitrary nature of the indicators that are characterised by the relatively scant attention that they pay to clinical outcomes. A trust can have excellent clinical results yet fail on other politically driven technicalities. The ratings are used to suit several different purposes and their use for purely political ends can result in unwarranted condemnation on an NHS trust that is derived from one brief snapshot view of limited aspects of its performance. While the system may be a useful tool for the Department of Health, it must certainly be confusing to patients who have experience of first-class care who find their local hospital is branded a failure. Claims have been made that the rating system has improved care. This, though, is a controversial issue according to many prominent commentators who doubt the veracity of the exercise (Kmietowicz, 2003a). This was further compounded by the allegation that political interference had occurred in the 2002 rating exercise whereby the ratings of some trusts were changed due to ministerial involvement, with the result that a hospital within the constituency of Tony Blair was a beneficiary and received three-star status (Mooney, 2004). What seems certain, however, is that evaluation within the NHS is here to stay, be it of this kind or of something more sophisticated.

THE COMMISSION FOR HEALTHCARE AUDIT AND INSPECTION (CHAI)

This body was established in April 2004 and immediately titled itself the Healthcare Commission to differentiate itself from its predecessor body the CHI. It is an independent body that operates at arm's length from government but reports directly to Parliament on the state of health care in England and Wales. It also acts as a means to rationalise the work of the several other regulatory and inspectorial agencies within the NHS that were created by New Labour. It is in effect a super-regulator with a brief to:

- Accelerate improvement in patient care and health care value-for-money across England and Wales.
- Strengthen the accountability of those responsible for the commissioning and delivery of health care.
- Demonstrate to the public how the additional money being invested in these services is being spent and enable them to judge how performance is improving as a result.
- Streamline NHS regulation by absorbing or co-ordinating the work of the following organisations:

- Audit Commission;
- Commission for Health Improvement;
- National Care Standards Commission;
- National Patient Safety Agency;
- National Clinical Assessment Authority;
- Commission for Patient and Public Involvement in Health.

The early promise of the new Commission was that it would be less dogmatic and more focused in the way in which it intended to handle its work than its forerunner (Donnelly, 2003). The initial plans of CHAI were that its visits to service providers would not be so standardised as its predecessor and should serve different and more specific purposes. These could be diagnostic, when information suggests there is a problem; confirmatory, to ensure initial conclusions are valid; facilitative, to support service enhancement; or random, in the form of spot checks made without warning to confirm or refute information that has been supplied to the Commission.

The director designate of CHAI gave early indications that the star ratings system would be abolished by 2006 and replaced by a new set of more generic indicators of performance (Kennedy, 2004). They were to examine not only performance achievements but also aspirational intentions of trusts and PCTs. This was followed swiftly by the launch of a public consultation on standards for better health that gave more scope for the independent CHAI to set standards rather than have them set politically (DOH, 2004b). This effectively marked a U-turn on the star rating system. The response from employee representatives was typified by the reaction of the BMA to this. It said:

> Doctors dislike and distrust the star ratings system. It serves only to measure the hospitals' ability to meet political targets and fails to recognise the quality of patient care. The process can interfere with patient care by skewing clinical priorities and neglecting the clinical needs of patients.
>
> We welcome a review of the system and hope the standards will not lead to yet another set of hoops for managers to jump through. Any new performance measures must be robust, transparent and meaningful. (Johnson, 2004: 1)

THE AUDIT COMMISSION

The Audit Commission is another public body responsible for ensuring that public money is used economically, efficiently and effectively. Its principal aim is to motivate the improvement of public services, oversee their proper stewardship and governance, and help those responsible for public services to achieve effective outcomes for users and the public by securing better value for money.

The Audit Commission has agreed a framework document with its sponsoring departments, and the Commission's Controller acts as its accounting officer. Its remit gives it access to all government departments, is far wider than the NHS, but its auditing functions in the NHS were transferred to CHAI for administrative convenience so that economic evaluations are under the same umbrella as other NHS inspectorial functions.

NATIONAL CARE STANDARDS COMMISSION (NCSC)

The National Care Standards Commission is an independent public body set up under the Care Standards Act 2000, to regulate social care and private and voluntary health care services throughout England. From 1 April 2002, the NCSC took responsibility for the registration and inspection of services by replacing the existing system of inspection by the 230 local and health authority inspection units. The following services are required to register with the NCSC:

- care homes and children's homes;
- domiciliary care agencies;
- residential family centres;
- voluntary adoption agencies;
- independent fostering agencies;
- private and voluntary hospitals and clinics;
- exclusively private medical practitioners;
- nurses' agencies.

In its first year of operation the NCSC claimed successful performance against its five objectives for the year in its mission to protect vulnerable people (NCSC, 2003). These were:

- 5,000 services were registered with the Commission;
- more than 50,000 inspections and visits were carried out;
- 100 per cent of registered adult services (23,000 services) were inspected;
- second inspections for all adults' and children's services assessed as high or medium risk: action taken on more than 12,000 complaints against services under its authority.

This new co-ordinated approach provided reassurance of an increasingly consistent, seamless and reliable system of regulation that had previously been both fragmented procedurally and of variable quality. The work began immediately to provide a wealth of information about the quality of services and the issues that face the social care sector.

NATIONAL PATIENT SAFETY AGENCY (NPSA)

The NPSA is a special health authority created in July 2001 to co-ordinate the efforts of the entire country to report on and to learn from adverse events that occur in NHS-funded care. As well as making sure events are reported in the first place, the NPSA strives to promote an open and fair culture in the NHS that encourages all health care staff to report potentially harmful incidents without undue fear of personal reprimand. It then collects information on reported incidents nationally and initiates preventative measures so that the whole NHS can learn from each case in order that patient safety can be improved.

The origins of the Agency are to be found in an expert report commissioned by ministers and chaired by the chief medical officer (DOH, 2000e). This stated that the NHS delivers a large volume of good quality care consistently. Yet the service had never had a formal risk management strategy despite undertaking activities that are known to contain hazards for patients. This had meant that things do go wrong, with serious and damaging consequences for patients and their families, that are almost predictable. The scale and nature of adverse events, and its huge cost was quantified by the report in stark terms that included:

- 400 people die or are seriously injured in adverse events involving medical devices.
- Nearly 10,000 people are reported to have experienced serious adverse reactions to drugs.
- Around 1,150 people who have been in recent contact with mental health services commit suicide.
- Nearly 28,000 written complaints are made about aspects of clinical treatment in hospitals.
- The NHS pays out around £400 million a year in settlement of negligence claims, and has liability of around £2.4 billion for existing and expected claims.
- Hospital-acquired infections – around 15 per cent of which may be avoidable – are estimated to cost £1 billion.
- Adverse events that harm patients occur in around 10 per cent of admissions – or at a rate in excess of 850,000 a year – and cost the service an estimated £2 billion a year in additional hospital stays alone, without taking into account human or wider economic costs.
- In addition, there is evidence that some specific types of relatively infrequent but very serious adverse events have happened time and again over a period of years.

- Inquiries and incident investigations determine that 'the lesson was learned', but the evidence suggests that the NHS as a whole is not good at doing so.
- Still less is known about the situation in primary care, despite the fact that it accounts for the great majority of NHS patient contact experience.
- Research in this country is in short supply and gives no indication of the potential true scale of the problem (DOH, 2000e: 1).

The report was at pains to emphasise that the NHS is not inherently negligent and that adverse events arise more from systems failure than from individual carelessness. Its authors found that the service did not learn from its mistakes for several reasons. They identified a blame culture that inhibited open reporting of things that go wrong where the energies of senior staff are concentrated on finding scapegoats in preference to studying how accidental occurrences might be prevented in the future. This in turn had led to a dearth of information that could be usefully shared to prevent adverse events from recurring.

The report concluded that greater transparency was needed to collect systematically the necessary intelligence about harmful or potentially harmful occurrences and to disseminate it more widely. Its authors felt also that the concept of the 'near miss' that is used within the aviation industry needed to be employed as a routine practice. This initial investigation gave way to a definitive risk management policy and the creation of the NPSA with clear direction to:

- Collect and analyse information on adverse events from local NHS organisations, NHS staff, and patients and carers.
- Assimilate other safety-related information from a variety of existing reporting systems and other sources in this country and abroad.
- Learn lessons and ensure that they are fed back into practice, service organisation and delivery.
- Where risks are identified, produce solutions to prevent harm, specify national goals and establish mechanisms to track progress (DOH, 2001b).

NATIONAL CLINICAL ASSESSMENT AUTHORITY (NCAA)

The NCAA is also a Special Health Authority and was established on 1 April 2001, following recommendations in reports made by the chief medical officer at the time of several high-profile cases involving medical malpractice, including the investigation and subsequent conviction of the serial killer Harold Shipman (DOH, 1999a and b, 2001c). Government was concerned that such incidents had begun to damage public confidence in the ability of the National Health Service and the medical profession to deal quickly, effectively and fairly with under-performing doctors. Although brought to light by the Shipman incident, other high-profile malpractice cases tended to be part of a pattern of poor medical practice that had developed over a long period of time. Of greater concern was that while the malpractice had occurred it had not been recognised officially. It was usually common knowledge within more informal local networks or had been discussed widely in professional settings. This confirmed that the long-established systems that might have been expected to detect problems had failed to do their job effectively and efficiently.

Further exploration revealed that the procedures that were in place for detecting and dealing with poor clinical performance were found to be fragmented and inflexible (DOH, 1999a and b). There was also evidence that some doctors who are performing poorly were not being confronted because employers were not willing to use the tortuous disciplinary procedures that were in existence. Such individuals were also difficult to hold accountable for their actions in some instances because of their seniority. Other professionals were therefore reluctant to report poor performance and, furthermore, procedures for dealing with complaints if they did arise were unwieldy and led to protracted and rancorous wrangling in expensive cases that diverted money away from treating patients. In consequence, patients were left vulnerable to poor practice and were not protected when they should have been. Equally, the under-performing doctors were also poorly supported when they needed to be.

Overall, government policy to strengthen quality assurance meant therefore that there was a pressing need to look more closely at the workings and regulation of the medical profession and address its deficiencies (DOH, 2001c). Concerns at the time focused on:

- Helping doctors to keep their skills and assuring the quality of individual practitioners through opportunities for continuing professional development and by the insistence that all practitioners submit to appraisal and to the clinical audit of their work.
- Protecting patients from adverse events by learning from failures of the past.
- Improving NHS-wide systems for quality improvement through the implementation of clinical governance by giving patients a stronger voice in their own treatment and in the management of the NHS. In addition, and as part of the review of quality improvement, NHS complaints procedures were reviewed and measures introduced for

checking the suitability of doctors at the appointment stage as part of improving public confidence in doctors.

- Factors to help those in practice included the creation of occupational health services and the provision of management training.
- Establishing the National Clinical Assessment Authority to better deal with doctors whose performance becomes sub-standard along with a review and standardisation of NHS disciplinary procedures.
- Monitoring the quality of NHS services locally through a systematic assessment of clinical governance by the Commission for Health Improvement (later the Commission for Health Audit and Inspection).
- Modernisation of professional regulation across all health professions with reform of the General Medical Council.

This wholesale examination of standards was interpreted by some as an attack on the medical profession, and the government was keen to offer reassurance that this was not meant to be. It stated that its intention was to, 'Reassure the public that regulation is being improved to protect patients and the public from the small but significant amount of poor practice which currently exists' (DOH, 2001c: para. 7.2).

Against this background of concern it can be seen that the NCAA represents the government's and the medical profession's shared commitment to supporting the principles of best practice, clear standards, high quality care and patient safety. It thus provides a support service to NHS primary care, hospital and community trusts, the Prison Health Service and the Defence Medical Services when they are faced with concerns over the performance of an individual doctor. The NCAA also provides support to the employers of hospital and community dentists about whom there are performance concerns. It is there to provide support to doctors and dentists in difficulty and to boost patient confidence in the NHS.

In order to help doctors and dentists in difficulty, the NCAA provides advice, takes referrals and carries out targeted assessments where necessary. The NCAA's assessment involves trained medical and lay assessors. Once an objective assessment has been carried out, the NCAA will advise on the appropriate course of action. The NCAA does not take over the role of an employer, nor will it function as a regulator. The NCAA is established as an advisory body, and the NHS employer organisation remains responsible for resolving the problem once the NCAA has produced its assessment.

COMMISSION FOR PATIENT AND PUBLIC INVOLVEMENT IN HEALTH (CPPIH)

The Commission for Patient and Public Involvement in Health and its place within consumerism in health care is considered in Chapter 3 (page 50), but it is worthy of exploration with regard to the Commission's regulatory functions. The Commission was set up in January 2003 and became operational in December of that year. It quickly abandoned its statutory title preferring the logo 'Shaping Health'. It also is an independent, non-departmental public body that is sponsored by the Department of Health and terms of reference concern direct public involvement in decision making about health and the provision of health services.

Section 11 of the Health and Social Care Act 2001 placed a duty on Strategic Health Authorities, Primary Care Trusts and NHS trusts to organise ways of involving the public in service planning, when considering proposals to change services and in seeking public views on the ways in which services are delivered and in assessing how well they are operating. These legal requirements were translated subsequently into policy guidance (DOH, 2003h). The duties given to the Commission intended that the way in which the NHS works will be open to public scrutiny and that it will be accountable more fully and formally to those local communities that it exists to serve. The CPPIH works in the belief that the patient experience should be incorporated into policy making wherever possible.

The Commission oversees and fully promotes the system of patient and public involvement. It establishes, funds, monitors and supports Patient and Public Involvement Forums (PPIF) and the delivery of the Independent Complaints Advocacy Services (ICAS). The Commission appoints members to the PPIF and ICAS and also provides guidance to them. The Commission is responsible for submitting reports to and advising the government on how the PPI system is functioning. It also liaises with national bodies such as the Healthcare Commission on patient and public involvement issues and makes recommendations to these bodies and the Department of Health as appropriate.

The Commission gathers information and opinion from PPI forums and channels this through its shared information system to ensure that the bodies to which it reports are acting upon patients' and the public's views. Its role in enhancing relationships between the service and the public has great potential in terms of standards concerning both acute and long-term care because it is acknowledged that many causes of patient dissatisfaction arise directly from poor communication by health service staff (Health Service Ombudsman, 2003).

It has been observed that public involvement in the NHS, though aimed at increasing democracy and responsiveness to patients, has grown in a piecemeal fashion (Florin and Dixon, 2004). The Commission therefore has a role to confirm where public involvement is at its most constructive and it forms a device for the NHS to use in evaluating itself.

THE MICRO-MANAGEMENT OF THE NHS: ITS ORGANISATIONAL CONTEXT

This chapter began by outlining how the NHS is controlled by a chain of command beginning with the secretary of state for health and how this is supported by the regulatory bodies that have been described so far. It will be seen, however, that the straightforward assumption that these formal structures guide and control the NHS in its entirety is wildly over-simplistic. They do have much to tell and they do contribute to its macro-management significantly. But there are aspects of its micro-management and control that are of equal importance to which the remainder of this chapter will be devoted.

Those at the sharp end are often not overly interested in the macro-management of the NHS for although it defines their day-to-day work they frequently feel remote from it. This is illustrated by the comments of a leading medical journalist when considering the then chief executive of the NHS: 'If he is the leader, then he's exercising a uniquely anonymous form of leadership. I doubt if one doctor in 50 could identify him' (Smith, 2003a: 1).

The micro-management of the NHS is a puzzle because of its compli-cated organisational composition and also because of the diverse vested interests that exist within it. This makes its management and control at a local level a difficult proposition. To achieve control of the NHS and to secure the particular wishes of policy makers, its management structures have received frequent and detailed attention. It has been reorganised 18 times in the last 20 years up to 2003, often in quite major ways. Each of these exercises has begun as a well-intentioned way of making it easier to control and better managed, the most recent example being the intro-duction of primary care trusts and the creation of foundation hospitals (DOH, 2001a). Yet the effectiveness of any one of these reorganisations is difficult to judge because most have never been thoroughly evaluated. What is known, however, is that most have had only minimal impact on some practices such as those of the medical profession.

Seeking better ways of controlling the NHS have resulted in it becom-ing increasingly more businesslike over the last two decades. The intro-duction of the notion of general management was introduced in February 1983 by the then secretary of state for health and social security, Norman Fowler. He had established an inquiry into the effective use of manpower and related resources in the NHS. A team led by Roy Griffiths, the then deputy chairman and managing director of Sainsbury's, presented its now infamous 25-page conclusions in a report about the inefficient leadership of the NHS that is summarised typically by the apocryphal quotation, 'In short if Florence Nightingale were carrying her lamp through the corridors of the NHS today she would almost certainly be searching for the people in charge' (DHSS, 1983: 24).

The Griffiths Management Review observed that NHS management at the operational level at the time, lacked logical consistency when judged against the sorts of standards employed in industry or commerce. Work measurement and evaluation systems were absent, performance targets concerning the setting and achievement of managerial objectives were obscure and there was little emphasis on customer care at all levels of the organisation. Accountability for clinical performance and the overall achievement and efficacy of the service were also found to be ill considered.

What followed from the report was to lay the template for the management system that exists currently, and its author recommended changes that have been implemented since the mid-1980s to increase central government control of even the remotest outer operational fringes of the NHS. The central message from Griffiths was to put individuals in charge through a system of general management that was to mark an end to the management by 'consensus'. General managers from within the NHS and from external commercial organisations began to be introduced. They were given clear levels of authority to devolve responsibility to their subordinates through a transparent structure of line management and through devolved budgets. Rigorous management training was initiated with a particular intention to arouse the interest of doctors in managerial matters. Stringent budgetary controls to avoid overspending were established and hospitals had to take on new forms of financial accountability. They were similarly charged to make efficiency savings that were reinvested to improve services. The introduction of this requirement to make efficiency savings led to an unprecedented emphasis on the achievement of better value for money by eradicating waste and increasing productivity. In effect, the drive was to get managers to provide more care and treatment from the same unit of resource.

The ambition of successive governments to better attract the medical profession into managerial posts saw painfully slow progress. A series of strategies failed to provoke their interest. Indeed, until the post-Griffiths era, doctors (whose clinical decisions are the precursor either directly or indirectly to most NHS expenditure) were only minimally responsible for the financial consequences of their clinical practices. The turning point came with the invention and spread of clinical directorates in the early 1990s. These comprised a series of semi-autonomous specialist directorates, each of which was led by a clinical director who was a senior consultant. Clinical directors were not meant to be line managers of all their staff but rather to act as persuasive leaders of those around them. They not only carried professional responsibilities for care but also were charged to agree with the general manager, the outputs to be achieved by their directorate through a specified level of clinical activity. This was linked to a predetermined budget and so, for the first time in the history of the service, doctors began to bear some responsibility for the financial consequences of their clinical decisions.

Prior to the Griffiths commentary on NHS management, the NHS was an administered organisation rather than one that was managed, and comparisons with private sector companies were regarded as somewhat invidious. Hospital administrators acted as passive diplomats to ensure a turbulence-free environment. They had few objectives to meet other than to stay in budget. The service was regarded as an essential public good that taxpayers were prepared to fund, irrespective of how much they used it. Its ethos was one of service rather than profit and because its outputs were considered to involve nebulous factors such as the quality of life, they were considered to be mainly unquantifiable.

What Griffiths had proposed was that the NHS had more in common with commercial organisations than had been supposed conventionally and that business practices were essential if its efficiency was to be improved. Sharp and assertive management practices were thus initiated to replace the previously passive administrative tradition that had been characterised by weak leadership, vague objectives, protracted decision-making processes, variable standards and very few outcome targets.

The Griffiths recommendations therefore brought a reorientation towards reduced bureaucracy, new forms of accountability and a new outlook that fuelled fresh approaches to customer care and patient satisfaction through the setting of standards. Initial comparisons with outside industry that regarded health care as a collection of commodities that were processed by the NHS and gave way to an end product could only, in reality, be partial for several reasons. The NHS is less transparent than most other organisations because what it does contains more that is unpredictable than for example, a production line operation, so therefore its product is less easy to define. Because it deals in high-risk matters as part of its task, complications in its business cannot always be predicted accurately. It also encompasses different professional vested interests within its workforce so that the adoption of corporate goals and a mutually shared identity is less easy to engender than in an organisation that manufactures a uniform and distinctive end product. Furthermore, the sort of economic sanctions that are experienced by failing companies are clearly inappropriate, and unsuccessful hospitals simply cannot be permitted to go into liquidation and to close their doors.

A further differentiation from commercial companies at the time Griffiths reported concerned the lack of incentives for major professional groups to improve their performance; a consequence of his work was the emergence of performance-related pay for senior managers, tied to the achievement of government objectives and attached to a rolling contract. The setting of detailed numerical performance targets and quality standards that have been described in Chapter 2 (pages 35–43) have reinforced the importance of these contractual arrangements for managers that are linked directly to the degree of success they have each year in meeting these specified goals, all of which are intended to yield greater output. In fact, managers of the most successful NHS organisations have been offered enticements to earn bonuses of up to 30 per cent of their annual salary, to bring their remuneration on a par with senior doctors, without whose co-operation success cannot occur (DOH, 2003i). The historically contentious aspects of performance-related pay systems concern, at a basic level, the presumption firstly of what constitutes good performance and, secondly, that it can be measured. Whilst an argument in its favour is that it motivates successful managers. Doctors, however, have resisted performance-related pay because they profess excellence and would not want any member of their ranks to be judged mediocre, poor or to be under-achieving.

MEDICAL POWER

THE LEGACY OF 1948

The medical profession has a rich history and as part of its agreed conditions of service when consenting reluctantly to join the NHS in 1948, it extracted a number of rights, concessions, freedoms and entitlements that have always rendered its position special (Foot, 1999). The profession of the day had become afraid of losing its autonomy and being transformed into an arm of the Civil Service. It was therefore only won over to signing up to the NHS at a price that it stipulated. The most well known of its indulgences are its contractual arrangements whereby GPs were, until the British Medical Association's acceptance of the piloting of the Personal Medical Services (PMS) Contract in 2000, mostly private contractors and were largely outside the NHS (DOH, 2003j). Despite the overall acceptance of this generous offer, those wishing to remain on a General Medical Services Contract (GMS) were permitted to do so and preserve their independence from the NHS. A new style GMS contract was unveiled for implementation in April 2004. This was intended to reward flexibility in the range of services that are offered and to provide additional payments for the delivery of high quality care that is based on the best available evidence. Yet both the PMS and the GMS contracts were not without their disadvantages to the service because many GPs exercise their right to decide, for only a small financial penalty, not to participate in out-of-hours work at evenings and over weekends. This leaves PCTs to cover the out-of-hours work by using expensive locum services or by re-engaging the same GPs who have opted out and wish to organise themselves in private co-operatives and set their own rates of reward.

At the inception of the NHS, hospital consultants were also given the liberty to conduct private practice alongside their NHS work and also, for most of the history of the NHS, they have controlled the usage of the greater part of its resources. This has focused the direction of spending mainly on sickness and on secondary care, and attempts to reverse this trend and empower primary care are relatively recent (DOH, 2001a). Throughout the life of the NHS, doctors' organisations have used twin tactics to accomplish and sustain their superlative status by lobbying and by threatening industrial action (Blane, 1997).

POLITICAL SUPREMACY

The medical profession therefore has skilfully ensured its political representation at every level of the NHS that matters to its interests. It does not need members of parliament to pursue its cause because, through the British Medical Association, its professional organisation and through its medical Royal Colleges, it has access to the ear of the chief medical officer and therefore a direct line to the secretary of state. Its power has led to the convention that any issue government intends to raise that is likely to be contentious with it is discussed with the profession prior to being made public. It has therefore endowed itself with the political muscle to be heard on any issue and to veto those things it finds unfavourable to it.

This overall political power has its origins in the 19th century that came as a reward for policing its own standards of professional conduct (Harrison et al., 1992). Its more local influence stems from the clinical authority that doctors have over all aspects of care and treatment, their control over patients, their influence of subordinate staff and their ultimate control over NHS output. All of this has been converted into a series of social roles by which the public generally perceives the profession. This centres on doctors as the sole repository of scientific knowledge about health and disease. Doctors' standing is further enhanced because their monopolistic tenure of skills concerned with the diagnosis and treatment of disease are enshrined in law and are not shared by any other professional grouping. The potency of health and disease as entities in the modern public psyche means that doctors command respect and, if they wish it, can demand deference. This is also reflected in their social status and in their high earning power. They are thus an authoritative source on any issue concerning health care that transcends their particular clinical expertise and they have a right to be heard on any policy or managerial issue in which they choose to take interest. Additionally, their political supremacy is bolstered by medical solidarity. For although the medical profession may quibble amongst itself, it unites strongly and is fiercely loyal to its own cause if it feels outsiders are threatening its territory. This does not mean that it is institutionally belligerent but it is exceedingly difficult to manage and to control if it is minded not to co-operate.

Managing the medical profession has therefore been a task taken on by successive governments over the last 20 years that have achieved only modified success in wresting power from it. The dilemma governments and for those charged with directing the medical profession face has been summarised as follows: 'Knowledge is power, knowledge management is the use of power for good' (Donaldson, 2003: speech to the National Patient Safety Agency, 18 March 2003).

This makes medicine by far the most powerful of all the professions in the NHS (Wilmot, 2003). Medicine has supremacy over other professions and carefully controls the content of their work that precludes other professions from doing anything other than tasks that it deems to delegate to them (Larkin, 1984). It has been similarly proposed that the medical profession's real control over resources makes it effectively the traditional owner of the NHS (Flynn, 1992). Its superordinate status has been described thus: 'The political truth is that the professions in health care include medicine, which retains a disproportionate degree of power and status; and the rest which do not' (Wilmot, 2003: 87).

DOCTORS AND MANAGERS IN THE MODERNISED NHS

During the first 40 years of the NHS the medical profession remained largely free from lay evaluation and maintained a dominant and omnipresent influence on all aspects of NHS life. It effectively defined the very nature of the service that was organised around its needs rather than those of patients. Clearly it was investigated if it was involved in overt negligence or illegality, but what surveillance of it that did exist had a light touch and was left to unstructured peer observations and the devices of its statutory regulatory body, the General Medical Council. The thought that others should manage medical activity did not occur to anyone.

The intrusion on medical sovereignty came stealthily with the evolution of managerialism that has been described as originating from the Griffiths Report, and this began to bite more seriously in the late 1980s and early 1990s. Doctors were brought into a new form of relationship with NHS managers as certain levers of control were given to the managers. Performance indicators had been introduced as a tool at the disposal of managers that gave crude evidence about the performance of consultant medical staff in hospitals that identified such things as the length of patient stay, throughput and turnover intervals for the first time. Consultants were scornful of this evidence because none of the measures provided any information about the actual clinical outcome for the individual patient. During this period, even less was known about detailed workings of general practice that was to remain relatively unmanaged for some time to come.

The document *Working for Patients* was published in 1989 and it introduced measures that potentially restricted the liberty of doctors by what, in theory, made them answerable to general managers (DOH, 1989). The report firmly stated a policy that clinical activity should be attached closely to the financial resources that were available. It became axiomatic, therefore, that consultant consent and co-operation were crucial to forging the link between the money that was to be had and their clinical work. The key element was to have a financial calculation attached to every clinical decision, although, at the time, pricing information was at its most primitive. This did, however, bring into stark contrast the variations in clinical practice and in the cost between clinicians, even for identical procedures and episodes of treatment.

Working for Patients also brought another innovation in terms of managing the NHS: it introduced the notion of medical audit. This gave managers a new responsibility for the quality of care through the power to oversee the conduct of individual doctors if it felt them to be practising poorly. Doctors who were wary, firstly, of the possible intrusion into their professional performance by lay people who lacked scientific training, treated this with general suspicion. Secondly, they feared that audit might lead to a position where procedures might be standardised through treatment protocols that could be designed by managers who were under pressure to save money (Flynn, 1992). Interestingly, consultants working in private practice in non-NHS hospitals have no complaint against treatment protocols specified by medical insurers, although they become an anathema when mentioned in relation to their NHS work.

Despite their apparent muscle in the doctor–manager relationship, managers were loath to act on their authority because of the imbalance of influence between themselves and the medical profession. For managers, it is not surprising that taking on the might of a profession that is apt to close ranks if it is challenged is not a risk that is worth taking in the interests of livelihood and career self-preservation.

It seems reasonable to conclude that medical independence remained fairly unscathed in the 1990s. Medical perceptions of managers and their posture towards them was influenced during the decade, as were medical attitudes to the NHS as an organisation, especially in terms of their improved awareness of the relationship between their clinical activity and the budgets of their directorates. The association between doctors and managers was one of benign toleration with episodic antagonism towards managers by doctors. The whole subject was to become far more inflammatory following the election of New Labour as clinical governance became obligatory and clinical services were restructured in direct opposition to the wishes of doctors (Pollit et al., 1997). Tensions were to intensify under the government's demand on managers to achieve political targets under the guise of modernisation, the *NHS Plan* and the barrage of new inspectorial agencies that were to accompany it.

Clinical governance was to become the principal instrument of surveillance of medical activity. It has been described as:

A framework through which NHS organisations are accountable for continually improving the quality of their services and safeguarding high standards of care by creating an environment in which excellence in clinical care will flourish. (Scally and Donaldson, 1998: 61)

Clinical governance reinforced managers' powers of policing medical performance. In effect this permitted managerial access to all aspects of medical autonomy (Harrison and Ahmad, 2000). This was described as comprising the following:

- control over diagnosis and treatment including the choice of techniques and drug regimes;
- control over audits of clinical performance;
- control over job plans and work measurement;
- contractual autonomy to engage at will in teaching, research, commercial consultancy and private practice.

In the past, medical activity attracted only scant attention in relation to its systems of clinical care delivery and it was left to the individual discretion of consultants to manage their time as they thought fit. Managing doctors have, however, become an international phenomenon resulting from the increasing cost of health care that requires managers to use resources more efficiently (Davis and Harrison, 2003). Understanding more about the detailed workings of the profession have also been stimulated by public reservations about medical accountability that intensified with the revelation of serious wrongdoing in high-profile cases of malpractice such as the Bristol inquiry (Stationery Office, 2001a). Nevertheless, it seems that although doctors have been resistant to managerial impositions they have eventually absorbed change and have not sought to put back the clock (Harrison and Lim, 2003).

THE CONSULTANT CONTRACT AND ITS IMPACT ON DOCTOR–MANAGER RELATIONSHIPS

The thought that medical work would be dominated even more fully by lay managers introduced new strain between them with the introduction by New Labour of a proposed new contract for consultant medical staff that sought to amend their conditions of service (DOH, 2002f). To pursue the *NHS Plan* and its modernising policies New Labour sought to limit the discretion of doctors even further through more detailed intervention by new impositions on the content of their work.

The *NHS Plan* had stated originally that the move to a consultant-delivered service would mean that, in the future, newly qualified consultants would be contracted to work exclusively for the NHS for perhaps the first seven years of their career by providing eight fixed sessions and more of the service delivery out of hours. In return, the government planned to increase the financial rewards to newly qualified consultants. The threat to private practice and the thought of being managed more strongly by lay managers led to intense acrimony. So aggravated were the consultants that they refused the offer made to them in October 2002 and they threatened to resign from the NHS *en masse*, arousing suspicions that they might move into chambers and sell their services to the NHS along the lines on which barristers operate (Garside and Black, 2003). Relationships between them and the then secretary of state, Alan Milburn, turned sour and it was only when he stood down from office that they accepted the concessions of his successor, John Reid, in June 2003.

This represented a climbdown by ministers, and differentials within the consultant contract were largely scrapped. The doctors accepted job planning but the priority in the exercise was shifted to allow for professionalism and the clinical judgement of consultants to decide job plans rather than have them determined by managers (BMA, 2003a). While consultants agreed to provide emergency care during evenings and at weekends, the original proposal that managers would prescribe this was also removed. Such cover was to become voluntary and consultants were to be rewarded at an enhanced rate for out-of-hours work they chose to do. The proposal was put to a vote of consultants and specialist registrars who were to benefit from the revised contract; the results are shown in Table 5.1. The proposals that were accepted provided some regularity to the conditions of service and gave a fuller account of the expectations NHS trusts would have of consultants. These are shown in Table 5.2.

Table 5.1   Beneficiaries of the revised contract

	Yes	Per cent	No	Per cent	Total	Turnout
Consultants	12,636	60.7	8,178	39.3	20,814	70.0
Specialist registrars	1,711	55.4	1,379	44.6	3,090	37.0
Total	14,347	60.0	9,557	40.0	23,904	62.0

Source: BMA (2003b)

Table 5.2 Benefits of conditions of service for NHS patients and consultants

Activity	Benefits for NHS patients	Benefits for consultants
Job planning	Improved ability to manage consultants' time to best meet local service priorities. Greater clarity of objectives for consultants and more effective engagement to improve NHS performance.	A stronger, unambiguous framework of contractual obligations. A more transparent framework for ensuring consultants have the facilities and support to carry out their responsibilities.
Working week and on-call duties	More efficient use of consultants' time contributing to NHS productivity and quality of care. Greater opportunity and incentives to deliver consultant delivered care in evenings and at weekends to give evening out-patient clinics and better emergency care.	More consistent and equitable recognition for on-call duties. Reduction of the number of consultants on the most frequent on-call rotas. More consistent and equitable recognition of work undertaken out of hours, including emergency work.
New pay structure	Improvements in recruitment and retention of consultants contributing to an increase of 15,000 consultants and GPs by 2008. Sustained incentives for high-quality performance over the course of a career. Enhanced incentives for consultants to maintain commitments for the NHS up to the age of retirement.	Increase of average earnings with final phase of consultant career rising by 24 per cent. Greater recognition of changing roles over an individual's working life.
Extra programmed activities	Ability to secure extra consultant activity more cost effectively.	Opportunity to undertake extra work on a more regular and predictable basis for the NHS.
Private practice	Preventing conflicts of interest between private practice and NHS commitments. Stronger guarantees that private practice will not detract from NHS performance.	Preventing unfair perceptions of abuse in relation to NHS consultants with private practice commitments. Abolition of maximum part-time contract and replacement with an NHS contract based on agreed time and service commitments.
Clinical excellence awards (England and Wales)	Greater scope for recognising outstanding performance. Improved quality of care through more transparent links between consultant reward and quality of service.	More equitable system of rewarding commitment and quality. Access to increased level of local reward for improving services. Consultants making the most outstanding contribution to receive £150,000 per annum.
New disciplinary arrangements (England only)	Faster, fair and more effective disciplinary procedures.	Faster, fair and more effective disciplinary procedures.

Source: DOH (2003j)

The furore over the consultant contract in 2002/03 compounded medical concerns over top-down, politically led policy making, budgetary controls and the target culture that prevailed. These factors served to emphasise that medicine and management are culturally different (Degeling et al., 2003; Smith, 2003b). In two separate analyses of these cultural differences and of the hostility between doctors and managers it was claimed that:

- Medicine is founded on more robust intellectual precepts than management, which contributes to its superior status.
- Medicine works at the bedside with real people and is answerable to them.
- Management and medicine hold disparate interpretations of responsibility and leadership that result, in part, from their occupational socialisation resulting in doctors not seeing the need to be led and not embracing the overarching organisational needs of the NHS.
- There is a need for both of these highly committed groups to form a consensus about the boundaries of clinical imperialism and its impact on resources that can only be achieved through mutual acceptance and collaborative working.

CONCLUSION

It can be seen from this chapter that the NHS is a complex organisation in terms of its size, its tasks and its professional cultures. Incrementally, over two decades, stronger management has sought to fortify the hold of managers over clinical activity by securing the greater accountability to them of 'hands-on' frontline staff by curtailing their clinical freedom and specifying the ways in which they will work. They have had success in this respect by determining the content of the work of nurses, midwives and therapy professions. Managerial control has been reinforced in more recent times with systems of inspection and surveillance.

While it is undeniable that there is greater accountability of the medical profession than previously, it still occupies a dominant and compelling place because of the power it has over the organisation through its monopoly of skills, significance of the decisions that it has to take, and the overall political power these convey to it.

The following chapter will assess the possibilities for health policy and for the direction of the NHS in the future.

SIX

THE UNFOLDING TALE

This chapter will look at the shorter-term future for the NHS and for health policy by returning to consider more fully some themes that were introduced in earlier chapters. It will then proceed to provide a broader account of the options that might arise to provide health care in general as the decade progresses.

THE SHORTER-TERM AGENDA

The achievement of the *NHS Plan* and the legacy of what was launched in 2000 will be a challenge for governments of any particular political persuasion in the years to come simply because of the magnitude of change set in motion by New Labour in both its first and second terms of office (DOH, 2000a). In a comprehensive review of the implementation of the *NHS Plan*, the Audit Commission identified a number of policy priorities for the Department of Health to address (Audit Commission, 2003b). It noted the likely difficulty that the service will face in meeting the targets it has set for older people and for those designed to improve its mental health services. The Commission observed the emerging and urgent management needs of primary care trusts (PCTs). Auditors were concerned that NHS trusts should be helped to demonstrate and record that new money has been spent to boost the services for which it was intended. Alternatively, if they have to be permitted to spend new money as they chose, then the parameters of their freedoms needed to be described in detail. Auditors also questioned the absolutist nature of the 'star rating' awards and suggested that trusts' true strengths as well as their weaknesses should be identified properly. Trusts in trouble were considered by the auditors who pointed to the need for their managers to look beyond blaming a lack of resources as the excuse for poor performance. The auditors felt that these trusts should concentrate on achieving greater efficiency and on improving the robustness of their financial recovery plans. Management capability was also highlighted with advice that poorly performing trusts should be linked to successful ones in a management mentoring arrangement that could become a function of the new NHS foundation trusts.

TARGETS OR STANDARDS?

The Audit Commission report also questioned the burdensome volume of targets, the preoccupation with waiting times and whether it was preferable to focus the closest attention on a much smaller number of priorities. This suggestion was reinforced by the House of Commons Public Administration Select Committee (HCPAC, 2003a). It identified the positive outcomes of performance measurement and of league tables and saw these as vital to both providing incentives to NHS organisations and to quantifying improvements. In this respect the Committee believed the government's intentions to be commendable. This constructive contribution to the improvement of publicly funded services was seen to provide:

- greater accountability;
- open information to the public and Parliament;
- a common definition of acceptable standards;
- valuable information to improve performance.

The Committee also expressed some reservations and saw the need to rationalise the number of performance targets within the public services generally as the mainstay of the system of performance measurement. It identified what it regarded as quite specific failings of the target-setting culture that concerned:

- lack of clarity about what the government is trying to achieve through the choice of arbitrary forms of measurement that sometimes lack credibility;
- failure to give adequate direction to those who provide services who are resentful that only headline targets receive publicity;
- failure to measure the right things leading to perverse consequences and sometimes even to cheating;
- failures in reporting and monitoring performance;
- confused accountability.

The Committee produced a highly critical review of the way in which public service achievements and failures were presented by government and about the degree to which these had become politicised. It observed that political parties' use of spin and that the use of arithmetical sleight of hand was hindering rational discussion about important areas of performance. The solution was seen in seeking independent, trustworthy corroboration through rigorous research and evaluation. Ministerial claims indicated that targets were contracting, yet paradoxically the Committee believed their range was being extended and that frontline staff were becoming demoralised by targets. Its report made the point that service users should contribute to the determination of what is desirable. It noted that local staff were using their ingenuity to dodge targets or outwit the target setters on occasions and it concluded that they also should be given fuller ownership in deciding what is possible when targets are being set.

It has been observed that performance monitoring in the public services is productive if it is done well but that it can be costly, ineffective and even damaging if it is done badly (Royal Statistical Society, 2003). In a rigorous scrutiny of current approaches to target setting and performance management it has been observed that performance indicators should be treated as a screening device and not as something to be regarded as an unassailable truth. It questions the methodological rigour of procedures that are in use and cites poor objective setting, concern for cost effectiveness in the design of procedures and a realistic estimate of the burden they will produce and involvement of those under scrutiny in the process along with constant safeguards for their dignity (Royal Statistical Society, 2003).

The issue of meeting targets is linked inextricably to capacity, which requires hospital beds to be available immediately an episode of treatment is considered to be completed. This raises another perpetual problem, namely that of delayed discharges. On any given day it has been estimated that there are 3,500 older patients in NHS beds in acute hospitals after medical staff have declared them fit to leave (HCPAC, 2003b). This occurs for the straightforward reason that their discharge arrangements are unfinished and this leads to a cost to the NHS of £170 million a year. The finding is highly pertinent to relevant targets to reduce waiting times because the inefficiency overall consumes 1.7 million lost bed-days and prevents other patients from receiving appropriate treatment. Although most of these delayed discharges are of short duration, about one-third exceed 28 days. These statistics question the feasibility of meeting government targets to reduce delayed discharges to around 3,000 by the end of 2004 and between 2,000 and 2,500 by the end of 2005. Clearly it is the most fragile and susceptible elderly who wait longest due to delayed assessment, lack of care home placements, problems with transfers for additional NHS care or delays in the availability of local authority services.

At the root of the problem, therefore, is the inefficient synchronisation of services, and improved co-ordination is needed between NHS acute trusts and its associated caring agencies. Introducing fines against local authorities who are adjudged responsible for delayed discharges was brought in under the Community Care (Delayed Discharge) Act 2003 to create an incentive for local councils to assess and arrange community care services for patients without delay. It seems, however, that this is unlikely to improve the way forward while ever there is the poor harmon-isation and poor partnerships between local authorities and the NHS. Diminishing government funding to support care home residents also aggravates the problem of delayed discharges. Furthermore, social service departments are often reluctant to put elderly people into care homes because in many instances, immediately a person without private means is admitted, social services have to meet the cost.

A conflict between the purpose of the delayed discharges legislation and the spirit of government policy to reduce disadvantage to the elderly and provide wider personal choice has been identified (Rowland and Pollock, 2004). Fines accrue to social services in effect if they have not made discharge arrangements within two days (DOH, 2003k). Official government policy is that patients will have choice over when, where and how they are to be treated and of greater choice of care at the end of life (DOH, 2003l). Yet within the context of declining capacity in social care accommodation, there is the speculation that far from having choices extended, older and chronically ill people may be misplaced on the grounds of expediency without having any say in the matter (Rowland and Pollock, 2004).

FOUNDATION HOSPITALS

The Health and Social Care (Community Health and Standards) Bill 2003 marked the beginning of what could be the break-up of the nationalised health services in Britain (Bosanquet and Kruger, 2003). A total of 130 backbench Labour MPs who signed a motion opposing the Bill, the centrepiece of which was the creation of foundation hospitals, supported this view. The protest of Labour MPs was also endorsed vociferously by the trade unions who complained that the development had not appeared in the manifesto, and had been subject to no consultation with patients, the community or staff (UNISON, 2003). The concerns that the trade unions had about foundation hospital status have been rehearsed in Chapter 3 (page 58), that it is regarded as being not so much about a new localism in health provision, rather it concerned a backdoor form of privatisation (Pollock, 2003). For while government policy portrayed foundation trusts as 'not-for-profit' organisations, their potential business freedoms suggested this might be far from the case. Despite New Labour's promise to retain foundation trusts as part of the NHS family, to have them accountable to local communities and to have independent regulation of them, their level of self-determination to raise private capital and to contract with private providers suggested the exact opposite. The misgivings about privatisation for those detracting from the ideology behind foundation hospitals was exacerbated by the way in which the Department of Health had canvassed private health providers who were lined up to bid for failing NHS trusts. Indeed, there was suspicion that the regulator for the new organisations would be under pressure to change the operating licence of trusts in financial difficulty to allow them to sell off assets and to accept private patient income (Kmietowicz, 2003b). The apprehension of MPs was shared by the Foundation Trust Concern, a coalition of 15 organisations representing doctors, therapists and major health unions under the co-ordination of UNISON. It summarised what it saw as the decision to allow the best performing hospitals to become foundation trusts, independent bodies with freedoms to set wages and attract private funding (UNISON, 2003). The organisation believed that foundation trusts would:

- Compete as part of a commercial market and PCTs will buy services from a range of different providers across the public and private sectors, including NHS trusts, foundation trusts and privately owned providers.
- Be a sly route to privatisation by allowing private and voluntary organisations to apply for trust status.
- Be poor value for money due to private borrowing that costs more than if they borrowed from the public sector.
- Lead to greater inequalities between hospitals, because foundation trusts would have greater powers and freedoms than NHS trusts, which will lead to inequalities in the health service.
- Poach scarce staff away from non-foundation trusts by offering better wages.
- Undermine the NHS public service principles by weakening integrated health services and reducing access to care.

Against this pessimistic interpretation was a contrasting view that foundation hospitals are a positive advance capable of inducing unprecedented improvement into health care (Bosanquet and Kruger, 2003). This was argued to stem from the establishment of an external market that by 2008 could see all hospitals liberated at least theoretically, from direct state control and to possess wide powers of autonomy in which the use of private funding can flourish. This thesis suggests that foundation trusts would leave behind the traditional ills of low productivity by producing a vibrant health economy. The 'two-tier' argument was rejected by advocates for the move because ultimately all hospitals would have foundation status. This contrasted markedly from the initial intention to grant the freedoms only to the elite high-performing trusts that had a 'three-star' rating. Rather than fragmenting care, the supporters believed that foundation status would revolutionise its delivery through new partnerships and alliances between primary and both public and private secondary care providers, voluntary agencies, social services and patients through much more care in community settings. In short it was contended that the legislation that paved the way for foundation trusts did not go far enough. It should, the protagonists believed, have included foundation standing for primary care trusts, and that 'profit' rather than 'not for profit', should have been a word in the vocabulary of both types of organisation (Bosanquet and Kruger, 2003).

PAYMENT BY RESULTS

The NHS financial reforms announced in the Budget of 2002 provided the largest ever sustained increase in NHS funding that was to be introduced over the succeeding five years (HM Treasury, 2002b). This amounted to 7.4 per cent real growth per year and set the course to match the European average spending on health care by 2008 that was discussed in Chapter 4 (pages 71–3). Assuming that the economy could continue to sustain this investment, which is dependent on its overall strength, the next challenge was to ensure that the extra money was used wisely in ways that demonstrate value for money is being realised. New Labour's safeguard in this respect was the economic model it chose to employ to fund health care from 2005 that also acts as something of a rebuttal to the critics of its foundation hospitals plan (DOH, 2003m).

Throughout the 1990s, budgets were usually a function of managers' negotiating skills and were arguably inconsistent and, on occasions, were patently unjust. Money was allocated on the basis of block contracts for packages of work. But the turbulence and fluctuation in activity sometimes left trusts under-rewarded for their actual endeavours. The rationale for revising the method of financial flows coincided with the objectives of the *NHS Plan* to produce a more personalised service, create high national standards with clear accountability and initiate greater local ownership of the NHS. All of this was designed to encourage innovation, increase flexibility for frontline staff and ultimately to extend choice for patients through greater diversity of provision. New Labour denied that its proposals for financial flows were a refashioned version of quasi-competition and of the former internal market of the Conservative Party years. It argued, rather, that it had produced a system of payment by results that is crucial to the success of a devolved health system where care is delivered by a diverse range of providers that is receptive to patients' needs and choices.

The advantages of these funding plans were claimed to be several. PCTs would be enabled to commission effective services that are more responsive to patients, produce a fair level of remuneration for providers and an even-handed price for commissioners. It follows from this that NHS trusts and other private and voluntary providers were to be paid fairly and transparently for services they would deliver and, because payment would be by results, the system intended to reward efficiency and effectiveness. This in turn would support greater patient choice, more finely tuned services and make a sustainable impact on waiting times. This idea would, in the future, therefore enable PCTs to concentrate on quality and quantity of the care that they purchase rather than what had happened previously, where the focus had been almost exclusively on its price.

The new financial arrangement was to depend on a tariff system of fixed prices, set by the Department of Health, that eventually would apply to care and treatment irrespective of where it was to be carried out. The tariff would relate more specifically to case mix than anything hitherto and would replace local price setting that had been so unpredictable nationally. The new approach overall was intended to act as an alternative to a totally free market where prices find their own level and was meant to invalidate accusations that privatisation was happening by stealth. The tariff system began to be introduced incrementally in 2003–04 when 15 health care resource groups (HRGs) were encouraged to bid for additional resources to support elective activity that related largely to other waiting time initiatives. Activity outside of the HRGs continued to be funded at a locally agreed rate. The pace of change was set to accelerate as HRG-related tariff funding increased to coincide with the advent of foundation hospitals. This meant that by 2004–05, 33 HRGs would be identified, making a total of 48 for which growth would be funded at tariff rather than locally set rates. By 2005–06 it was planned that almost all specialities would be commissioned on a cost and volume basis that would be adjusted for case mix. This marked a timetable to move away completely from locally set prices with its replacement by a nationally set tariff.

The funding plan ensured that patients would bring funding with them in a much closer way than previously and commissioning arrangements were to exist to properly monitor performance and also to provide incentives that reward excellence where providers were able to demonstrate it. The success of this considerable cultural change would depend on the sophistication of the pricing system that demanded skilful accountancy to properly generate knowledge about labour costs that perhaps did not exist when the financial flows plan was invented (Plumridge, 2003). In competitive terms, NHS organisations seemed vulnerable from the outset to external providers who had latitude to open up niche markets that were certain of a good financial return. These niche markets would be profitable because they would be fashioned around care pathways that are used in private medicine elsewhere in the world.

The unveiling of the detail concerning the tariff system aroused suspicion from its critics with the claim that this effectively reintroduced the market into the NHS, seven years after Labour pledged to abolish it (UNISON, 2004). The real criticism centred around the claim that the scheme is intended to extend to treatments bought from the private sector by 2008 with the warning that in some cases the health service was paying up to 50 per cent more for operations in the private sector than the same procedures would cost if they were carried out in NHS hospitals. It was further alleged that the private sector would build up an enormous advantage over NHS hospitals, some of which may be forced in the future to go out of business and to close. The corollary of this was seen to be that once the private sector became the only alternative it would increase its prices even more (UNISON, 2004).

As well as ideological criticism of the tariff system there was also that of a practical nature (BMA, 2004). While supporting the overall notion that money should follow the patient, it was suggested that no system is sufficiently sophisticated to take account of all the factors for those who go into hospital for a simple operation that leads to the NHS having to deal with a range of other related problems that will not be covered by the tariff.

It was predicted, therefore, that some tariffs would be far lower than the real costs of providing care, putting undue pressure on hospitals to make cuts.

MARKET FORCES

While there was a formal denial from government that there was to be any return to market forces, the proposed system of financial flows was meant undoubtedly to operate on the basis of competition. Foundation trusts would need to compete for patients and although, as has been observed, the criteria for recruiting business would be on quality criteria rather than price, competition would be inevitable. The extent to which competition can bring genuine benefits for health care has been debated extensively (Dixon et al., 2003). The conditions for stronger competition at the creation of foundation hospitals were far better than they had been in 1991 when the Conservative government introduced the internal market. This was so because the objectives of consultants and managers had become more resonant than they were then and, furthermore, consultants were to be given monetary inducements to do more work that were not available when competition was introduced originally. Set against this were the unfavourable aspects of market competition that result in activity being focused on the profit motive. This could work to the detriment of those patients, often with chronic illnesses, who are the least lucrative than, say, those needing elective short-term interventions. An interesting prognostication concerning competition and market forces worthy of consideration was depicted as follows:

> Perhaps a 'fork in the road' is now possible, with elective (surgical) care provided by competing hospitals, and other forms of care stimulated by more appropriate incentives. New conceptions of 'market' in the NHS may emerge – allowing more vertical integration between primary and secondary care providers. (Dixon et al., 2003: 5)

CLINICAL GOVERNANCE AND QUALITY IMPROVEMENT

It has been seen from Chapter 5 (page 107) that New Labour, as the principal mechanism for assuring quality care, introduced clinical governance progressively as a means to improving public confidence in the NHS and the concept was also adopted by other non-NHS providers (NHS Executive, 1999). This came out of the recognition that, although financial and workload targets were very evident, that quality did not have similar primacy within NHS thinking. Clinical governance became obligatory and led to the assembly of procedures to control overall aspects of quality and to include risk-management strategies, adverse incident reporting and the provision of better information for patients. The measures provide benchmarks that form the basis of the institutional assessments of trusts that were conducted from 2004 by the Commission for Health Audit and Inspection and used for the performance rating methodology.

In a landmark report by the National Audit Office (NAO) to Parliament, that assessed the consistency of clinical governance arrangements, it was revealed that progress showed variation both within individual trusts and between them (NAO, 2003b). The audit identified much good practice and noted the way in which the orderliness of clinical governance was producing more explicit accountability from managers and clinicians as well as encouraging a culture that fostered team working. While changes had been developmental and had concentrated necessarily on establishing processes, clinical governance had produced important attitude change.

This was leading towards the shared and transparent acceptance of responsibility between trust executives and clinicians and was producing palpable progress in developing patient services.

Yet the report's reservations about patchy performance were several, and included the following:

- clinical audit was reportedly irregular with only half of trusts claiming its use in more than 80 per cent of its clinical directorates;
- adequate resources to sustain the various elements of clinical governance were deficient along with low participation in training events about it;
- the prevailing culture continued to inhibit the reporting of risks;
- patient centredness through the involvement of users and the general public was considered to be underdeveloped.

There were obstacles to progress that were acknowledged to be beyond the control of individual trusts. Developments such as mergers and the organisational complexity this sometimes produced had brought the pursuit of contradictory objectives. This arose from attempts to achieve such factors as short-term waiting targets was also an unavoidable hindrance to some trusts.

In its recommendations, the NAO recognised that clinical governance was in its infancy and that good progress was evident. In sustaining the impetus, the report recognised the significance of the Modernisation Agency's Clinical Governance Support Team in encouraging trusts and in propagating best practice. It called also for the appraisal of schemes that were being devised to engage patients and the public in governance so that the parameters of the best systems could be defined and publicised widely. It was suggested that trusts themselves should regularise and streamline their reporting systems on clinical governance to their trust boards.

After this encouraging analysis the future task presumably became one of nurturing shared governance. This would require an even greater change of culture whereby traditional hierarchical relationships would be replaced by all staff becoming equally engaged in a multi-professional strategy of quality enhancement (Burnhope and Edmonston, 2003).

The success in raising the profile of quality of care that the NHS has enjoyed through clinical governance was also indicative that it was achieving its intention of becoming a learning organisation (DOH, 1999b). Such organisations have been defined as follows: 'Learning is something achieved by individuals, but "learning organisations" can configure themselves to maximise, mobilise and retain this learning potential' (Davis and Nutley, 2000: 998).

Such organisations adopt techniques to manipulate their internal culture by appealing positively to commonly held beliefs (Mintzberg et al., 1998; Davis and Nutley, 2000). Techniques that are employed to bring about a learning organisation include:

- Acknowledging attainment and high achievement to reinforce its value to the organisation.
- Seeking continuous improvement through a commitment to novel solutions and rejecting any idea that the status quo is ever adequate.
- Learning from mistakes by avoiding a blame culture and accepting that it is possible to learn from adverse events.
- Valuing the contribution of all, however seemingly insignificant, and seeking to expand their career opportunities.
- Acknowledging intuition and the value of what individuals know through personal and practical experience.
- Creating transparency through free channels of formal and informal multi-professional communication.
- Having faith in individuals and giving them the confidence and the facilities to act independently and to experiment in the knowledge that management will support them.
- Knowing what happens elsewhere in other professional communities both within the organisation and in similar organisations elsewhere.

It can be seen that becoming a learning organisation is an ambitious undertaking that requires a long-term transformation in its cultural norms. Despite a lack of formally accrued evidence there are signs from the NAO report that the task was begun in the NHS.

PATIENT CHOICE

It will have been seen from previous chapters that patient involvement has become a major plank in the modernisation agenda for the NHS. Despite a long history of seeming to involve patients in their own health care, progress has been slow with 'expert'-driven care remaining the norm. It has been acknowledged, however, that patients with chronic disease can become important decision makers in the management of their condition and have useful contributions to make to service planning (DOH, 2001d). There have, however, been changes in significant trends concerning social status and social identity of senior professionals in the NHS (Pietroni et al., 2003). It has been observed that over the last 60 years there has been:

Loss of deference towards figures in authority
Knowledge explosion through popular books, media, and internet
Rise of consumerism and focus on patients as customers
Rise in litigation and downfall of doctors as heroic figures
Rise of managerialism that challenges professional hegemony.

(Pietroni et al., 2003: 1304)

There is, nevertheless, recognition and indeed compelling evidence that giving patients choice puts pressure on doctors and on other professionals. While the public want more say in choices about their care and treatment, both they and their GPs were worried about the impact that providing choice would have on the workload of family doctors (BUPA/MORI, 2003). In a survey that recruited a representative sample of the general public and GPs it was suggested that 88 per cent of doctors and 46 per cent of the British public were apprehensive that extending patient choice would put more pressure on GPs. Another concern was indicated by 75 per cent of the public who admitted to being puzzled by the amount of contradictory health advice that was available to them. The same proportion relied on their GP to interpret the confusing array of information for them. Furthermore, 38 per cent of the general public sample believed that NHS patients currently do not have any choices and an additional 36 per cent 'don't know' what choices are available to them.

These findings also indicate that as well as fearing the burden of pressure on their workload, GPs consider patient choice equates to better standards of care. This differs from the anticipation of the public, only 46 per cent of whom considered the opportunity to express a preference would confer better care. There were other more surprising conceptions about choice between GPs and the public. GPs thought that 75 per cent of patients would want a say in the selection of a surgeon but only 40 per cent of the public felt they should determine this.

Both samples had some qualms about the issue of choice, yet both thought it should be offered and that patients should pick which hospital they preferred. GPs also supported a view that patients should be given fuller details about their therapeutic regime.

Despite the mutual support for choice in these findings there was much to suggest that the entire notion of patient choice is subject to multiple interpretation. It is likely that asking health care professionals what patient and public involvement means to them can provoke antagonism from those that oppose the idea and irritation from those who think that they have always involved the patient (Pietroni et al., 2003). This raises the interesting possibility of having professionals who are trained to involve patients and the public through the shift from 'doing to' patients to 'doing with' them in the creation of sustainable public involvement.

THE PATIENT'S PASSPORT

The Conservative critique of New Labour health policy concerned the ultimate flaws it sees in the NHS (Duncan-Smith, 2002; Conservative Party, 2003a). These can be summarised as:

- its central control from Whitehall has become discredited;
- the monolithic structure is inefficient and wasteful;
- politicians, not clinicians, dictate decisions and the NHS only responds to political demands rather than patients' needs;
- bureaucrats and obsession with artificial targets guarantee power will remain with central government;
- the patient has no choice;
- there are no enticements for most staff to improve their performance.

The Conservative response to this would be to depoliticise the NHS and give power to the professionals and to patients by responding to their choices. The Conservative Party argued therefore that truly authentic choice is only available to those who not only pay tax but who also have private health insurance (Conservative Party, 2003b). Their pledge to introduce a Patient's Passport was intended to make choice an entitlement for the entire population. The passport would be used to pay for treatment in the NHS or as part or wholly funded treatment in the private or voluntary sector. The cost would be reduced for anyone with private insurance or for those willing to pay from their savings, and this was intended to extend the uptake of private medical insurance in terms of personal and occupational schemes. The plan was predicated on hospitals being removed from political control, and employing a national tariff system of the sort that has been described on pages 116–18 where activity is funded according to the volume of work completed and where, through patient choice, new private providers would be attracted into the market place (Conservative Party, 2003a).

New Labour's response to the Patient's Passport was predictable. It forecast that the Conservative Party was committed to destroying the values of the NHS, notably through the removal of equal access to health care regardless of ability to pay (Reid, 2003). It reiterated its commitment to the original values of the NHS and its commitment to equity and indeed claimed it had set up the National Institute for Clinical Excellence to see fair treatment of all. New Labour believed consensus about the NHS had been established for 60 years and that, consistently, three-quarters of the British people agree that the NHS is critical to British society and wish to do everything to maintain it. Public satisfaction with the NHS was allegedly at its highest for 10 years and as a social issue it was more important than any other including crime and immigration (Reid, 2003).

New Labour claimed that as the NHS gets better, private medical insurance gets dearer. British people reject private insurance, the uptake of which New Labour believed to be in decline, not because the people are unwilling to pay but because they recognise the inequity its introduction would cause.

The Conservative Patient's Passport was seen by New Labour as a means to the dissolution of the NHS and as a voucher scheme where people who can afford to pay for private operations would be subsidised to the tune of 60 per cent of the cost by using money intended for the NHS. Those who could not afford to pay the 40 per cent cost towards their operation in the private sector would be left waiting in a queue until their name came to the top of the waiting list. New Labour regarded the Conservative Party's one and only firm spending commitment on health to be a costly and bureaucratic plan. Its opposition included the claim that to subsidise those with the wealth to pay privately would cost £1 billion per annum. Furthermore, the reintroduction of tax relief on private medical insurance would, according to New Labour, take money out of the NHS and put it into the pocket of the richest people in the country with private medical insurance (Reid, 2003).

LOOKING FORWARD

IMPROVING THE PUBLIC HEALTH

It is a universal experience that health care is becoming more complex. Pathologies are changing and the interactions between nature, nurture and lifestyle are infinitely more convoluted than was imagined previously (Plsek and Greenhalgh, 2001). This means that interpreting the origins of good health and the aetiology of disease by using the faulty machine model has become intellectually unwieldy. To understand health and disease it is increasingly apparent that the interface between biological, psychological, cultural, behavioural and socio-economic factors are all compelling considerations (Bartley et al., 1997). The NHS was born when the epidemiological remnants of the diseases of poverty such as infectious diseases were the principal concern. In the present day the diseases of affluence predominate yet their distribution among the socio-economic classes has changed very little despite almost 60 years of a comprehensive NHS with the less well off having disproportionately more premature morbidity and mortality (DOH, 1998b). This has serious implications for policy makers, for although the post-war welfare state did not have a specific public health agenda at its core, its impact on life expectancy is equivocal. The main beneficiaries of this have been the non-manual and skilled manual classes with the least skilled fairing worst. There remain areas of the country where life expectancy is no more favourable today than it was in 1950 (DOH/HM Treasury, 2002).

One of the first things New Labour did on coming into office was to commission an independent inquiry into inequalities in health (DOH, 1998b). That inquiry report provided the firm foundation of evidence needed about the nature and scale of health inequalities. The *NHS Plan*, which had been luke-warm on the overall state of the public health initially, proceeded to recognise these inequalities and identified a 10-year programme for tackling them through the more effective prevention and improved primary care that was to be aimed at disadvantaged populations (DOH, 2000a). This long-term view was supplemented by an interim three-year programme to address the disparity in infant mortality across social groups and raise life expectancy in the most disadvantaged areas faster than elsewhere (DOH, 2003d). Such proposals recognised the obdurate nature of health inequalities both in their origins and in terms of doing something effective to alleviate them. New Labour therefore took on an ambitious task that centred on the geographical, ethnic and socioeconomic disparities that are known to be so resistant to change.

The multifactorial nature of the problem of health inequalities was restated. An action programme was produced to embrace the interventions of secondary care that accepted the value of direct therapeutic interventions through preventative drug treatments such as statins to reduce cholesterol and influenza prophylaxis by vaccination. But it observed also the significance of improving nutrition and increasing levels of physical activity in reducing instances of cardiovascular disease, diabetes and some cancers. The task was acknowledged to be too immense to be tackled solely by the NHS. This would require the mobilisation of many other participants including volunteers, businesses, service users, carers and community groups (DOH, 2003d). The crucial need for co-ordination across government departments was also rightly recognised through the contribution of other wider-reaching initiatives, including the following:

- *Sure Start* – this is a joint programme conducted by the Department for Education and Skills and the Department for Work and Pensions that aims to increase the availability of child care, improve the health, education and emotional development of young children, to support parents in their role and to further develop their employment aspirations.
- *National Strategy for Neighbourhood Renewal* – this strategy operates under the auspices of the Office of the Deputy Prime Minister and sets out the government's vision for regeneration by narrowing the gap between deprived neighbourhoods and the rest of the country so that

within 10 to 20 years no-one should be seriously disadvantaged by where they live.

- *UK Fuel Poverty Strategy* – is a Department of Trade and Industry initiative formulated to support housing improvements and to conserve energy that is targeted at vulnerable households.

Added to these were measures to increase employment opportunities, the national minimum wage, welfare and benefit reforms, transport and housing improvements and educational changes that all became part of the strategy to reduce health inequalities.

The Department of Health and the Treasury jointly conducted a cross-cutting review to assess progress in reducing health inequalities and to get a consensus on the priorities for future action (DOH/HM Treasury, 2002). This gave way to a long-term strategy to reduce health inequalities through a cross-government delivery plan that traversed traditional departmental boundaries. This valiant plan aimed to disseminate responsibility to the core of every key public service in a concerted action to harness and direct the strength of billions of pounds towards the reduction of health inequalities (DOH, 2003d).

Both the socio-economic dimension and the more health-specific aspects of health inequality were targeted within this strategy that identified the activities it believed likely to have greatest socio-economic impact over the long term. These were:

- improved support for young children and families;
- improved social housing and reduced fuel poverty among vulnerable populations;
- improved educational attainment and skills development among disadvantaged populations;
- improved access to public services in disadvantaged communities in urban and rural areas;
- reduced unemployment, and improved income among the poorest.

More specific health-related targets to maximise the impact on known determinants of the life expectancy gap were:

- reducing smoking in lower socio-economic groups;
- preventing and managing the other known risk factors for coronary heart disease and cancer through effective primary care and public health interventions, especially targeting the over-50s;
- improving housing quality by tackling cold and dampness, and reducing accidents in the home and on the road;

- tackling inequalities in infant mortality – key short-term interventions included:
  - improving the quality and accessibility of antenatal care and support for children in socio-economically deprived areas;
  - smoking cessation and improved nutrition in pregnancy and improved nutrition for young children;
  - preventing teenage pregnancy and supporting teenage parents;
  - improving housing conditions for children in disadvantaged areas.

In attempting to improve the health of the poorest fastest, the Tackling Inequalities Action Programme was organised around four themes that reflect the foregoing analysis of the root causes of inequality (DOH, 2003d). These concerned:

- supporting families, mothers and children to ensure the best possible start in life to break the vicious intergenerational cycles of poor health;
- engaging communities and individuals to ensure the relevance, responsiveness and sustainability of health promotion programmes;
- preventing illness and providing effective disease treatment by making certain that the NHS provides adequate leadership and makes the contribution to reducing inequalities that is expected of it;
- addressing the underlying determinants of poor health by dealing with the long-term underlying causes of health inequalities.

This programme was unique in the history of the NHS both in its extent and in the intended sophistication of its organisation. It aimed at strategic goals, the success of which would not be evident for years to come but that confront one of the more unyielding obstacles within prospective health care.

The need to close the gap in health standards between the more affluent and the less well off was further emphasised in the interim report into population health trends (HM Treasury, 2003). It observed Britain to compare unfavourably with other comparable Western countries in terms of mortality and morbidity across the socio-economic groups. The countries studied included France, Germany, Sweden, Denmark, Finland, the Netherlands, Australia and Canada, and the report suggested that the UK has much to learn from them in terms of its approach to maintaining the public health.

The UK had the highest infant mortality rate and relatively high mortality from cancer and coronary heart disease. In 2001 England had 5.5 infant deaths for every 1,000 live births, compared with 3.1 per 1,000 in Finland. Respiratory disease resulted in the deaths of 135 men in every

100,000 people in England, the highest proportion of all the countries, compared with 50 men per 100,000 people in Sweden.

The investigation called for a better understanding and insights into the social aetiology of health that include diet, exercise, housing and employment. It concluded that if action were not taken to reduce inequalities within the next 20 years, the projected cost to the NHS would require an additional £30 billion each year to cope with the consequence.

RADICAL NEW DIRECTIONS FOR HEALTH POLICY?

There are shades of opinion which hold that despite New Labour's occupation of the Conservative Party's customary terrain, it still had not gone far enough in reforming public policy (Browne and Young, 2002; Reform, 2003). Reform is an independent campaign to promote new directions for public policy based on the principles of free enterprise, limited government and individual liberty. In a report by its Commission on the Reform of Public Services it alleged that Britain has the poorest public services of any other comparable developed country (Reform, 2003). It disputed vigorously that, despite additional investment, New Labour had not reformed the NHS conspicuously. The report cited the source of the problem to be national prosperity. This it saw at one level as being dented by punitive tax increases that reduce the motivation and the productivity of individual citizens who have no incentive to work harder if it means they will be taxed still further than they already are. The hindered position of individuals within the economy is further compounded by the progressive escalation of government spending on the public services that diverts investment away from a private sector that is capable of yielding higher productivity. The outcome is seen as inferior services that work to the detriment of the most disadvantaged who get the poorest treatment and care.

The report considered Britain to be ready for radical change in the way its public services operate currently (Reform, 2003). This was to be accomplished by transferring spending power from the government to individual citizens who would be liberated to act as individual consumers. Providers of services would thereby be given the necessary encouragement and latitude to provide exactly what consumers want. Flowing from these underlying principles were specific recommendations for the NHS, as follows:

- The attempt to provide NHS services through collective responsibility should be abandoned. Individual patient choice should drive health care provision.
- The NHS should become a purchasing agency only with money directly following the patient to provider organisations that would be outside NHS control.

- Two funding options were proposed. One would grow progressively from a tax-funded system to become ultimately fuelled by private health insurance in its entirety. The second would be more uncompromising still and would see an instantaneous introduction of private health insurance.

A similar far-reaching proposal examined the nature of alternative funding systems for health care (Civitas, 2002). It described what it saw as the system that was suited ideally to be the source of funding for British health care. The report believed that the government's role should be confined to that of a regulator and that its responsibility for health care should be limited to the creation and maintenance of a legal framework for services to be provided. In consequence, government would withdraw from the day-to-day political control that would pass to clinicians. Patients would have freedom to select where and when they are cared for and providers would vie for their custom under marketplace conditions. There would be no compulsory user payments because private insurance would be obligatory.

There is, therefore, a further view that the policy to create foundation hospitals is a half measure that falls short of the sweeping change needed to exploit the opportunity more fully by transferring possession of all hospitals to 'not-for-profit' community trusts (Civitas, 2003). The report of a consensus group comprising different hues of Labour Party political opinion that included clinicians, concluded that the opponents of foundation hospitals were unrepresentative of modern-day socialist thinking. In preserving the intention to maintain universal access to health care, this treatise maintained that only a minority of the most rigid socialists remain committed to communal action of the type on which the NHS was established. This belief stems from contact with social democrats in Europe who, unlike the British, are perfectly content that hospitals be controlled by non-governmental organisations and where there are no qualms that anyone who needs treatment will get it irrespective of their financial circumstances (Civitas, 2003). The report argued that:

- Ownership of all hospitals should pass immediately from government to 'not-for-profit' community-owned and community-controlled organisations on the assurance that they would be used exclusively for the provision of health care.
- Hospitals would be allowed to raise whatever private capital they wished and this would not be a liability to the taxpayer because their management bodies would be required to relinquish any claim to public funds.

- One safeguard to the access to treatment would be that emergency care and treatment would be available to all.
- In being liberated completely from government control, these new institutions would be empowered to make their own conditions of employment.
- Any new hospitals could be built and 'for-profit' providers would be permitted to enter the market.

The report considered the ownership of hospitals once they pass out of state control and considered how they might exist as independent legal entities (Civitas, 2003). Their initial autonomous status would be 'not for profit' with their assets preserved for the benefit of the public and these would be prevented from passing to private hands. Four models of tenure were considered feasible that fell short of full-scale 'for-profit' shareholder-owned privatisation on ethical grounds. These were as follows:

- *Mutual societies* – these are co-operatives or provident societies that function as 'not-for-profit' organisations that do not have shareholders but are owned by their members.
- *Charity status* – this would resemble the status of some hospitals prior to the foundation of the NHS and the institutions would register with the Charity Commission and their assets would not be allowed to pass into private hands.
- *Charted status* – this model would function on the lines of British universities whose authority is specified by the Privy Council through a Royal Charter. Their rights cannot be amended without the approval of the Council and their assets cannot be used for private purposes.
- *Lease Model* – under this arrangement the government would continue to own hospitals but would lease current NHS building stock to either 'not-for-profit' or to 'for-profit' organisations.

It can be seen that radical ideas to break the mould in which the NHS was cast originally are both plentiful and contain some intellectual consistency in seeking to apply new values that are in direct contradiction of the old and fixed policy prescription for health services in Britain. The advent of New Labour has made it, at the very least, receptive to transformational policies for health care. The extent of what is possible is, as ever, a matter of political feasibility. This relates partly to the party political implications of radical NHS change in mid-term and its possible impact on a future general election. New Labour, however, considered itself so well insulated politically that it has left itself room for manoeuvre. This was justified by its claim that the NHS was only truly safe in its hands because the Tories were pledged to 'destroy' the health service (Brown, 2003).

Politically significant also, were the internal dynamics of the Labour Party that retained sufficient vestige of 'Old Labour' socialist support to make a truly reforming government have to think twice before tinkering with the NHS. The arguments against change were two-fold. Firstly, the existence of the NHS is living proof that the welfare state is intact. Any attempt to meddle with its fundamentals is likely to be interpreted by time-honoured opinion as a deliberate attempt to extinguish it. Secondly, there is the contention that in retaining the NHS as it is, there is a predictability about it and Britain knows what it can expect. In contrast, the more drastic alternatives that have been outlined have not been tried and tested. This renders them high risk, requiring further testing and valuation before they could be considered as serious alternatives to what exists.

INTO THE DISTANCE

There is a growing literature of interest to policy makers that has attempted to anticipate the demands of health services as the next decade progresses (Warner et al., 1998; Dargie et al., 2000). These are variously attributable to a range of factors from the increased availability of new technology and scientific advances, to the effects of globalisation, to global warming and to food safety that demand the attention of policy makers.

MORE ELDERLY PEOPLE TO CARE FOR

Some of the predicted trends are already evident and there are others that remain within the realm of speculation. In terms of Britain, it is possible to anticipate the demands for health services of an increasingly ageing population, especially those over the age of 80 years. This will bring epidemiological changing trends in patterns of morbidity with an increase in age-related degenerative disease and malignancy that are the accompaniments of longevity. Patterns of care will inevitably alter to give far more care at home requiring many more ageing informal carers and a far greater reliance on social systems to maintain the well-being of elderly people. The NSF for Older People represents a significant policy that recognises and anticipates these forthcoming health and social care needs (DOH, 2001a, 2002g). The framework was developed with advice from an external reference group comprising older people and their carers, health and social services professional staff, NHS and social services managers, and partner agencies. It provided a plan and a set of standards to eradicate age discrimination and make certain that older people are valued appropriately and with dignity. It seeks to have older people maintained as independently as possible by a well-integrated, well co-ordinated, coherent approach to the assessment of individual need. This is intended to be met by services tailored specifically to the hazards and illnesses of later years such as falls, deteriorating cognitive abilities and strokes. The framework also showed cognisance of prevention through its intention to promote the health and well-being of older people through co-ordinated actions of the NHS, local authorities and voluntary agencies. Progress with the implementation of the programme was to be monitored through a series of milestones and performance measures that are overseen by the NHS Modernisation Board. Its creation also provides the milieu for further systematic study of ageing processes and strategies for their amelioration and management.

WHO WILL PAY?

Paying for health care in Britain in the future will remain a challenge. There will be a need for a sustained strong economy to uphold existing plans to increase NHS spending. But as the birth rate remains low and the numbers of people in paid employment that sustain the current taxation-fuelled system decline, there will be compulsion to look at alternative sources of funding. The argument that it is unfair that those in work should pay taxes to sustain public services that they do not use is a recent phenomenon. This originated through the debate about tuition fees for university students and provided what may become a large wedge within the welfare state landscape that was rehearsed by New Labour, as follows:

> Of course the taxpayer will – quite rightly – always pay the lion's share. But I believe that it is reasonable and fair to ask graduates to pay a proportion of the costs of the university education from which they benefit for the rest of their life. (Clarke, 2003: speech to the Labour Party Conference)

Parallels of this philosophy were denied as far as the NHS is concerned but there is an ominous feel about the future viability of a largely tax-funded health service despite the optimism of the findings provided by Wanless (HM Treasury, 2002a).

QUALITY AND THE INFORMED CONSUMER

Society is changing and factors such as increased personal wealth at one end of the economic scale and residual poverty at the other will make the policies to alleviate inequalities in health and in life expectancy a continuing test. A better-informed public with new rights, choices and entitlements as consumers add to the task. Most will be computer literate and have access to self-diagnosis to add to their authority as consumers. This can be calculated to erode the monopoly on knowledge that was once in the gift of professionals who will have to serve a more discerning, assertive, safety-conscious and more involved public.

The NHS has begun to anticipate this through its various attempts to address quality and performance, and disseminate information about best practice that were addressed in Chapter 5 (pages 87–99). The criticism that customer care and satisfaction are ill-considered is no longer a valid assertion, although the scope for choice to which the NHS aspires is perhaps more difficult to attain than has been assumed. It is likely, nevertheless, that the quest for improvement will continue relentlessly and that quality in the NHS will be exposed more publicly for the benefit of local patients and strategically through international comparisons of its performance (Dargie et al., 2000). New Labour showed a commitment to transparency of performance and the reduction in its variation from place to place and this mission will become more highly developed at the local level. In terms of international comparisons, there has always been the criticism that these are unreliable because of the different ways in which data on the performance of health services are collected internationally. The OECD, however, is providing solutions to this by the generation of health data covering a wide range of policy-relevant topics ranging from population health status to the non-medical determinants of health care resources that will be needed and their utilisation. Data are also collected on health insurance coverage and on health care within overall social care systems. In approaching this intricate assignment, the OECD health data team works not only on a regular data collection process but also provides statistical support for policy analysis. In addition, it also acts as a source of methodological advice on health statistics that guides the design of national health information systems and has established benchmarks that permit international comparisons. By deciphering emerging issues and identifying policies that work, it therefore helps policy makers by informing their strategic orientations.

UNLIMITED TECHNOLOGY

The expansion of new technologies in health care is unstoppable and the scope for their therapeutic impact is boundless. Yet each new discovery raises questions about its cost effectiveness. Britain is long past the time when it could afford all the technology at its disposal, and studied decisions have to be made. The NHS is entering an era of unprecedented challenge to the accepted role of service provision and professional practice and will continue to focus on the indices of excellence and on influential scholarly debate about innovation and quality enhancement.

NICE exists to provide guidance for health care professionals, patients and their carers that inform their decisions about treatment and health care. It provides independent authoritative advice about the use of new and existing health technologies such as medicines, medical devices and procedures, the management and care of specific conditions through to the production of clinical guidelines and in the use of new surgical techniques. The Institute also disseminates information learned from deaths and adverse events involving technology. The real test of its virility are the occasions when it has been moved to recommend the implementation of technologies that were thought previously to be prohibitively expensive that have resource or political implications that government is unable to ignore.

CONCLUSION

This book has attempted to provide a pragmatic appraisal of health policy in Britain at the start of the 21st century by exposing both the multifaceted nature of the subject through the dilemmas and the tensions that face policy makers. Medical technology and social policy in Britain have developed in largely separate ways and their fusion is a relatively recent phenomenon, and is in no small measure due to the policies of New Labour. The predicament has loomed large between national priorities and local imperatives and this will remain. This requires respectful conciliatory co-operative working to solve it. Allocation issues will continue also to puzzle policy makers and these can be examined on several axes.

HEALTH SERVICES VERSUS OTHER SERVICES
NHS spending is in competition with other demands on government that include, prominently, defence, education, law and order, roads and transport. At the inception of the NHS ill health was a priority. Yet almost 60 years on most people live to be old and, for most, medicine is not a factor in their survival. In addition, they rarely use the NHS substantially until after their retirement. This raises a question about the relative importance of spending on health and who should bear the brunt of it. Health spending in Britain has been accepted conventionally to be a collective responsibility, yet health services are used for the vested interests of individuals. This has led to the orientation that suggests individuals might take more

personal responsibility for their own health care by making a financial contribution to it through, for instance, private health insurance. This in turn might engender a more health-conscious self-caring population.

PREVENTION, CURE AND PALLIATION

An obvious thought with regard to getting best value for money from health spending is that it would be a good investment to engage in more prevention. It might also be assumed that screening for more conditions is a possibility. There is, however, a strong and embedded intellectual custom that prevention is difficult to measure and is therefore a less legitimate activity than treating established disease where success and failure are easier to quantify. It is a reasonable assumption that there is the possibility for both more prevention and more effective therapeutic interventions but there will always remain the manifestations of ageing. Illness has also become very much a social process that is concerned with the discharge of obligations and with the fulfilment of a social role. There is therefore a case for directing attention towards the social antecedents and accompaniments of disease as well as to the technologies to treat it. Policy has been legitimately shaped by technology, and only recently with New Labour's interest in public health have broader realities been acknowledged officially.

HOSPITAL VERSUS NON-HOSPITAL SERVICES

A notable feature of recent health policy has been the intended transfer of purchasing power and responsibility away from the secondary care sector (DOH, 2001a). Primary and social care may be more desirable to individual patients. But these are not necessarily cheaper than hospital care if the quality is to be maintained, as has been illustrated by experience with the wholesale transfer of the mentally ill to the community. The test for the future of community care lies in the drawing of more effective plans for chronic disease management of the sort that has been embarked upon by the National Service Frameworks (NSFs). These are beginning to set national standards and identify key interventions for a defined service or care group, devise strategies to support their implementation, establish ways of measuring progress within an agreed time-scale to raise quality and decrease variations in service.

DOCTORS VERSUS OTHER PROFESSIONALS

Doctors are unequivocally the leaders in managing life-threatening illness. Yet in an era of chronic disease there is scope for a yet unrealised contribution from others. Care of the sick is no longer the sole prerogative of the medical profession that calls for multi-professional alliances. This will inevitably result in increasing changes in the allocation of responsibility and in opportunities and in the reward of other professionals.

During its illustrious history the NHS has often lacked a clear rationale, and its objectives have thus been blurred. Medical technology has appealed to the masses and has led the direction of the service irrespective of its cost or its efficacy. The modern New Labour era has seen a transformation that, although heavy-handed in some respects, has created a new decisive direction and purpose for the NHS that confronts reality head-on.

GLOSSARY
TERMS USED IN RELATION TO NHS POLICY

Audit Commission – the Audit Commission is the public body with responsibility to see that public money is used economically, effectively and efficiently, whose functions regarding the NHS were incorporated into CHAI in 2004 (www.auditcommission.gov.uk/).

British Medical Association (BMA) – the BMA is the main labour relations organisation representing doctors (www.bma.org.uk/ap.nsf/Content/_Home_Public).

Cabinet Office – is the personal Office of the Prime Minister that exists to co-ordinate activity across government departments, an activity that is known colloquially as *joined-up government* (www.cabinetoffice. gov.uk/).

Central command and control – the strong influence of health ministers over local health management primarily through the setting of rigorous performance targets but sometimes by direct intervention in local management decision making.

Commission for Health Audit and Inspection (CHAI) – CHAI was established formally as an independent body in 2004 to rationalise and co-ordinate the work of other regulatory and inspectorial organisations that oversee the NHS. It is known colloquially as the Healthcare Commission to differentiate it from its predecessor body (www.chai.org.uk/Home page/fs/en).

Commission for Health Improvement (CHI) – CHI was an independent body created to inspect the NHS in terms of its clinical governance systems, the achievement of its major delivery targets, its quality and in its implementation of evidence-based practice. It was absorbed by CHAI in 2004 (www.chi.gov.uk/).

Citizenship theory – a social theory underlying the relief of need that guided the introduction of the welfare state in Britain.

Clinical governance – the strategy and procedures governing quality, clinical audit, risk management and better information for patients in the

NHS and other health service providers that is intended to sustain public confidence in the NHS.

Commission for Patient and Public Involvement in Health (CPPIH) – the CPPIH was created as an independent, non-public body in 2003 that exists to ensure direct public involvement in decision making about the NHS and in the provision of its services (www.cppih.org/).

Community Health Councils (CHCs) – CHCs represented the broad community interest in NHS services from 1974 to December 2003 and were replaced by the Commission for Patient Involvement in Health.

Consultant Contract – the agreement on consultant delivered services reached in 2003 that provided a fuller account of the expectations NHS trusts could expect from their consultant medical staff through mutually agreed job plans.

Consumer/user – the contemporary definition of individuals in contact with NHS services. In its orthodox form, consumers make rational, informed choices in their best personal interest on the basis of their own evaluations of the alternative options.

Department of Health (DOH) – the DOH is the policy-making hub of the NHS that is based in Whitehall (www.doh.gov.uk/).

Equity principles – the principles of fairness on which the NHS was founded.

Foundation hospitals/NHS foundation trusts – independent, publicly funded hospitals with wide commercial freedoms that were introduced from 2004 and are subject to independent regulation.

Free market – a system of exchange that is powered by the price mechanism and relies on free competition and a contractual relationship between suppliers of goods and services that, at its extremes, means the strongest competitors make profits and their weakest counterparts become insolvent.

General Medical Services Contract (GMS Contract) – the GMS Contract is the terms of service provided for GPs who retain their independent contractor status and exercise control of what services they wish to provide that is known colloquially as the *Red Book*. A new style GMS contract was unveiled for implementation in April 2004. This was intended to reward flexibility in the range of services that are offered and to provide additional payments for the delivery of high quality care that is based on the best available evidence (www.doh.gov.uk/gmscontract/implementation.htm).

General taxation – compulsorily deducted taxation at source, paid largely by those in employment but from which the retired with personal savings are not exempt that is known colloquially as PAYE (pay as you earn).

Gross domestic product (CGDP) – the GDP is a measure of the strength of the economy; the percentage of the total of GDP that is spent on the NHS is used as a measure of the adequacy of health service funding.

Health Professions Council – an organisation to oversee the work of professional regulation that is conducted by the General Medical Council, the Nursing and Midwifery Council and the Council for Allied Health Professionals (www.hpc-uk.org/).

Health Service Ombudsman – the Health Service Ombudsman looks into complaints made by or on behalf of people who have suffered because of unsatisfactory treatment or service by the NHS or within the private care sector where the NHS has purchased services. The Ombudsman is completely independent of the NHS and the government and the services provided are free to complainants (www.ombudsman.org.uk/hse/).

Hypothecated tax – an earmarked tax that has a part to play in funding the NHS through the National Insurance contributions of people in employment.

Independent Health Care Association (IHCA) – the IHCA is an organisation representing private hospital, nursing and care home providers.

Internal market – the purchaser–provider relationship for purchasing publicly funded health services that was introduced in 1990, has been modified since, but is still in use in a re-branded form.

Local improvement finance trusts (LIFT) – LIFT uses capital that is raised privately to upgrade GPs' premises.

Mixed economy – the provision of services using state and non-state sectors that include private, voluntary and charitable suppliers.

Modernisation Agency – an organisation created by the DOH in 2001 to provide strategic support for the implementation of the *NHS Plan* alongside strategic health authorities, primary care trusts and NHS trusts (www.modern.nhs.uk/home/default.asp?site_id=58).

Monetarism – the predominant economic doctrine in Britain since the 1980s that is also known as the quantity theory of money.

National Audit Office (NAO) – the National Audit Office scrutinises public spending on behalf of Parliament and is independent of government. It audits the accounts of all government departments and agencies as well as a wide range of other public bodies, and reports to Parliament on the economy, efficiency and effectiveness with which government bodies have used public money (www.nao.gov.uk/).

National Clinical Assessment Authority (NCAA) – the NCCA was established in 2001 to help doctors maintain their skills, contribute to the overall quality of medical practice and deal with sub-standard medical practice to protect patients (www.carestandards.org.uk/).

NHS Confederation – a body that represents NHS trusts collectively (www.nhsconfed.org/).

NHS Executive – the operational arm of the DOH that exists to implement its policy that is based in Leeds (www.nosa.org.uk/contacts/nhsexec.htm).

NHS Plan – a 10-year plan to modernise health care in Britain that was launched by New Labour in 2000 (www.nhs.uk/nationalplan/).

NHS trusts/trust – providers of largely hospital-based care. Mental health and ambulance trusts are the exception to this, the former supplying both hospital and community-based services and the latter, transport services.

National Institute for Clinical Excellence (NICE) – NICE was created to evaluate new medical technologies and drugs on the basis of their costs and benefits before their wholesale introduction and use in the NHS. The results are converted into guidelines that trusts are mandated to follow as part of the drive for evidence-based practice (www.nice.org.uk/).

New Labour – the post-1995 Labour Party led by Tony Blair that adopted a radical new version of policies that resembled those previously attributable to the Conservative Party (www.labour.org.uk/).

National Patient Safety Agency (NPSA) – the NPSA was created in 2001 to co-ordinate the risk management strategy for the NHS to enable it to learn from adverse events that occur in care and treatment (www.npsa.nhs.uk/).

New Right – an ideological persuasion that typified the governments of Margaret Thatcher, which emphasised the primacy of the individual, private ownership and freedom from state control.

Office of National Statistics (ONS) – the ONS is a valuable source of data about health care nationally (www.statistics.gov.uk/).

Old Labour – the traditional left wing of the Labour Party that supported socialist principles that fostered collective responsibility for all aspects of welfare.

Organisation for Economic Co-operation and Development (OECD) – the OECD is an organisation that represents the world's richest nations and collects internationally comparable data about the health services of its member countries (www.oecd.org/home/).

Overview and Scrutiny Committees (OSCs) – OSCs are democratically elected members of local authorities who are intended to scrutinise variations and developments in local NHS service provision.

Patient Advisory and Liaison Services (PALS) – PALS exist in every NHS trust to represent all aspects of patients' interests.

Patient's Passport – the Conservative Party's intended mechanism that would extend choice and reduce the political control of health services (www.conservatives.com/).

Performance indicators (PIs) – PIs are used to measure NHS inputs, processes and outputs.

Politicised NHS – the importance of the NHS at the ballot box.

Personal Medical Services Contract (PMS Contract) – the PMS Contract was agreed by the BMA in 2003 whereby GPs who wished it, could renounce their independent contractor status and would supply an inclusive range of services tailored specifically to the needs of the patients in their practice (www.doh.gov.uk/pricare/pca.htm).

Primary care trusts (PCTs) – it is PCTs that deliver primary care services and purchase 75 per cent of secondary care on behalf of their patients.

Private finance initiative (PFI) – the PFI uses privately raised capital to build public utilities such as schools, prisons and hospitals that are then leased back or mortgaged to the state. PFIs usually have four key elements that are design, finance, build and operate.

Private medical insurance/health insurance – contributions made wholly or partly by individuals or more usually in association with employers to cover the cost of private health care and treatment.

Public–private partnership (PPP) – a PPP is a contractual arrangement in which a private provider contributes wholly or in part to the delivery of services that were formerly provided publicly.

Royal Colleges – the bodies regulating post-graduate medical training of doctors that validate the award of fellowships in the various medical specialities. The exceptions to this are the Royal College of Nursing and the Royal College of Midwives that have an interest in continuing professional development of their members that are also labour relations organisations.

Select Committees – all-party specialist committees of the House of Commons that make judgements on government performance that are independent of the governing party of the day. The Health Committee is of particular interest (www.parliament.uk/parliamentary_committees/health_committee.cfm).

Social Insurance – the method of paying for health services in much of continental Europe.

Star ratings – the colloquial term for the intellectually contentious performance rating methodology that ranks provider organisations in the NHS according to their performance on a range of indicators that are conflated into a single score that awards three, two, one or no stars (www.doh.gov.uk/performanceratings/).

Tariff – the fixed price set by the DOH to be introduced incrementally between 2003 and 2006 that applies to a specific case mix known as health care resource groups (HCRGs), which would be paid by purchasers of health services for the delivery of treatment irrespective of where it is provided. It is intended that this will allow money *to follow the patient* more closely than previously. It also means that payment to trusts will be made according to the results they achieve (www.doh.gov.uk/nhsfinancialreforms/events.htm).

Third Way – a doctrine that guided the policy of New Labour that attempts to embrace old Labour beliefs in social justice but simultaneously employs free-market principles to secure its political ends.

UNISON – a major labour relations organisation representing NHS employees (www.unison.org.uk/).

Waiting times – the targets set by government to reduce delays in receiving medical consultation or direct treatment for NHS patients.

World Health Organisation (WHO) – it is the WHO that collects and disseminates information on the state of the public health internationally (www.who.int/en/).

OTHER REFERENCE SOURCES THAT ARE USEFUL FOR THE STUDY OF HEALTH POLICY

Adam Smith Institute (www.adamsmith.org/).

Association of Chief Executives of Voluntary Organisations (www.acevo.org.uk/main/index.php?content=main).

Cochrane Library (www.update-software.com/cochrane/).

Centre for Policy Studies (www.cps.org.uk/).

Centre for Public Scrutiny (www.cfps.org.uk/).

Conservative Party (www.conservativeparty.org.uk/).

Dr Foster (www.drfoster.co.uk/).

Fabian Society (www.fabian-society.org.uk/int.asp).

Health Development Agency (www.hda.nhs.uk/).

Health Foundation (www.health.org.uk/).

HM Treasury (www.hm-treasury.gov.uk/).

Independent Health Care Association (www.iha.org.uk/).

Institute for Fiscal Studies (www.ifs.org.uk/).

Institute for Public and Private Policy Research (www.ippr.org.uk/home/).

Institute for the Study of Civil Society (Civitas) (www.civitas.org.uk/).

Institute of Economic Affairs (www.iea.org.uk/).

Institute of Healthcare Management (www.ihm.org.uk/).

Kings Fund (www.kingsfund.org.uk/).

Laing and Buisson (www.laingbuisson.co.uk/).

Liberal Democrat Party (www.libdems.org.uk/).

NHS Alliance (www.nhsalliance.org/).

New Health Network (www.newhealthnetwork.co.uk/).

Nuffield Trust (www.nuffieldtrust.org.uk/).

Office of Health Economics (http://195.200.28.182/ohe/ohehome.nsf).

Picker Institute (www.pickereurope.org/).

Policy Futures for UK Health (www.jims.cam.ac.uk/research/health/polfutures/polfutures.html).

Reform (www.reformbritain.com/).

Social Market Foundation (www.smf.co.uk//site/smf/).

Socialist Health Association (www.sochealth.co.uk/).

United Kingdom Parliament (www.parliament.uk/).

REFERENCES

Andrews, G. (1991) *Citizenship*. London: Lawrence and Wishart.

Appleby, J. (1999) 'Government funding of the UK National Health Service', *Journal of Health Service Research Policy*, 4 (2): 79–89.

Appleby, J., Harrison, A. and Devlin, N. (2003) *What is the Real Cost of More Patient Choice?* London: Kings Fund.

Audit Commission (2001) *Acute Hospital Portfolio: Review of National Findings – Accident and Emergency*. London: Audit Commission.

Audit Commission (2002) *Access to Care*. London: Audit Commission.

Audit Commission (2003a) *Waiting List Accuracy*. London: Audit Commission.

Audit Commission (2003b) *Achieving the NHS Plan Assessment of Current Performance, Likely Future Progress and Capacity to Improve*. London: Audit Commission.

Bartley, M., Blane, D. and Montgomery, S. (1997) 'Socioeconomic determinants and the life course: why safety nets matter', *British Medical Journal*, 314 (7088): 1194.

BBC (2000) Tony Blair's interview with Sir David Frost. *Breakfast with Frost*, BBC1, 16 January 2000. London: British Broadcasting Company.

Blair, A. (1998) *The Third Way. New Politics for a New Century*. London: Fabian Society.

Blane, D. (1997) 'Health professions', in G. Scambler (ed.), *Sociology as Applied to Medicine*. London: Saunders. pp. 212–24.

Blaxter, M. (1995) *Consumers and Research in the NHS: Consumer Issues within the NHS*. London: Department of Health.

BMA (2003a) 'BMA concludes talks on new consultant contract', press release, 17 July 2003. London: British Medical Association.

BMA (2003b) 'Consultant contract ballot', press release, 20 October 2003. London: British Medical Association.

BMA (2004) 'Tariff could cause problems says BMA', press release, 6 February 2004. London: British Medical Association.

Bodenheimer, T. (1997a) 'Oregon health plan – lessons for the nation – first of two parts', *New England Journal of Medicine*, 337: 651–6.

Bodenheimer, T. (1997b) 'Oregon health plan – lessons for the nation – second of two parts', *New England Journal of Medicine*, 337: 720–3.

Bosanquet, N. and Kruger, D. (2003) *Strong Foundations*. London: Centre for Policy Studies.

Brown, G. (2003) 'The NHS is only truly safe with us and our values', speech to the Labour Party Conference, Gordon Brown, Chancellor of the Exchequer, 29 September 2003, Bournemouth.

Browne, A. and Young, M. (2002) *NHS Reform: Towards Consensus*. London: Adam Smith Institute.

BUPA/MORI (2003) 'Can healthcare afford the informed consumer?' Results of a survey conducted for the British United Provident Association, London, by Market & Opinion Research International, London, September 2003.

Burnhope, C. and Edmonstone, J. (2003) 'Feel the fear and do it anyway: the hard business of developing shared governance', *Journal of Nursing Management*, 11 (3): 147–57.

Butler, E. and Pirie, M. (2001) *The New Shape of Public Services. Vol. 1: Health and Education*. London: Adam Smith Institute.

Butler, E. and Yarrow, G. (2001) *Welfare: A Research Agenda*. London: Adam Smith Institute.

Cabinet Office (2001) *Strengthening Leadership in the Public Sector*. Cabinet Office Performance and Innovation Unit London (www.cabinet-office.gov.uk).

Calman, K., Hunter, D. and May, A. (2001) *Things Can Only Get Better: A Commentary on Implementing the NHS Plan*, Durham: University of Durham Business School.

CHI (2003) *Getting Better? A Report on the NHS*. London: Commission for Health Improvement.

Civitas (2002) *Options for Funding. Interim Report of the Health Policy Consensus Group*. London: Institute for the Study of Civil Society.

Civitas (2003) *A New Consensus for NHS Reform. The Final Report of the Health Policy Consensus Group*. London: Institute for the Study of Civil Society.

Clarke, C. (2003) 'Education – always our priority', speech to the Labour Party Conference, Charles Clarke, Secretary of State for Education, 30 September 2003, Bournemouth.

Conservative Party (2003a) *Setting Patients Free*. Launch of a Conservative Health Consultation Document. London: Conservative Party.

Conservative Party (2003b) 'Patient's Passport', speech by Dr Liam Fox, Conservative Spring Forum, 16 March 2003, Harrogate.

Coulter, A. (2002) 'After Bristol: putting patients at the centre. Commentary: patient centred care: timely, but is it practical?', *British Medical Journal*, 324 (7338): 648–51.

Cox, K., Bergen, A. and Norman, I.J. (1993) 'Exploring consumer views of care provided by the Macmillan nurse using the critical incident technique', *Journal of Advanced Nursing*, 18 (3): 408–15.

Dargie, C., Dawson, S. and Garside, P. (2000) *Policy Futures for the UK. Health 2000 Report*. London: Nuffield Trust for Research and Policy Studies in Health Services.

Dash, P. (2004) 'New providers in UK health care', *British Medical Journal*, 328 (7435): 340–2.

Davies, C. (2003) 'Spell it out', *Health Service Journal*, 113 (5844): 31.

Davies, P. (2001) 'Trolley bad show dashes any lingering hopes. NHS plan targets are drifting further from being achieved on time', *Health Service Journal*, 111 (5779): 17.

Davis, H.T.O. and Nutley, S.M. (2000) 'Developing learning organisations in the new NHS', *British Medical Journal*, 320 (7240): 998–1001.

Davis, H.T.O. and Harrison, S. (2003) 'Trends in doctor–manager relationships', *British Medical Journal*, 326 (7390): 646–9.

Day, P. and Kline, R. (2002) 'Who nose best?', *Health Service Journal*, 112 (5799): 26–9.

Degeling, P., Maxwell, S., Kennedy, J. and Coyl, B. (2003) 'Medicine, management and the "danse macabre"?', *British Medical Journal*, 326 (7390): 649–52.

Deming, R.H. (1968) *Characteristics of an Effective Management Control System in an Industrial Organisation*. Boston, MA: Harvard Business School Press.

DHSS (1983) *NHS Management Inquiry Report*, chaired by Roy Griffiths. London: Department of Health and Social Security.

Dixon, J. and Harrison, A. (1997) 'Funding in the NHS: a little local difficulty', *British Medical Journal*, 314: 216–19.

Dixon, J., LeGrand, J. and Smith, P. (2003) *Can Market Forces be Used for Good?* London: Kings Fund.

DOH (1989) *Working for Patients*. London: HMSO.

DOH (1997) *The New NHS: Modern, Dependable*, Cmnd 3807. London: Stationery Office.

DOH (1998a) *A First Class Service: Quality in the New NHS*. London: Department of Health.

DOH (1998b) *Independent Inquiry into Inequalities in Health*. London: Department of Health.

DOH (1999a) *Supporting Doctors, Protecting Patients*. London: Department of Health.

DOH (1999b) *Continuing Professional Development Quality in the New NHS*. London: Department of Health.

DOH (2000a) *The NHS Plan – A Plan for Investment, a Plan for Reform*, Cmnd 4818-I. London: Department of Health.

DOH (2000b) *Delivering the NHS Plan: Next Steps on Investment – Next Steps on Reform*. London: Department of Health.

DOH (2000c) *NHS Implementation Plan*. London: Department of Health.

DOH (2000d) *For the Benefit of Patients: A Concordat with the Private and Voluntary Health Care Provider Sector*. London: Department of Health.

DOH (2000e) *An Organisation with a Memory: Report of an Expert Group on Learning from Adverse Events in the NHS*. London: Department of Health.

DOH (2001a) *NHS Shifting the Balance of Power within the NHS–Securing Delivery*. London: Department of Health.

DOH (2001b) *Building a Safer NHS*. London: Department of Health.

DOH (2001c) *Assuring the Quality of Medical Practice: Implementing Supporting Doctors, Protecting Patients*. London: Department of Health.

DOH (2001d) *The Expert Patient. A New Approach to Chronic Disease Management for the 21st Century*. London: Department of Health.

DOH (2002a) *Delivering the NHS Plan: Next Steps on Investment – Next Steps on Reform*. London: Department of Health.

DOH (2002b) *Growing Capacity. A New Role for External Healthcare Providers in England*. London: Department of Health.

DOH (2002c) *A Guide to NHS Foundation Trusts*. London: Department of Health.

DOH (2002d) *Involving Patients and the Public in Health Care*. London: Stationery Office.

DOH (2002e) *Prescriptions Dispensed in the Community. Statistics 1991–2001: England*. London: Department of Health.

DOH (2002f) *Consultant Contract: Framework*, November 2002. London: Department of Health.

DOH (2002g) *National Service Framework for Older People Meeting the Milestones*. London: Department of Health.

DOH (2003a) *Creating Responsiveness and Equity in NHS and Social Care. A National Consultation*. London: Department of Health.

DOH (2003b) *The NHS Plan. A Progress Report – The Annual Report of the Modernisation Board, 2003*. London: Department of Health.

DOH (2003c) 'Trust will review waiting times reporting systems', press release 2003/0092. London: Department of Health.

DOH (2003d) *Tackling Health Inequalities – A Programme for Action*. London: Department of Health.

DOH (2003e) 'Patient focus. Improving the patient experience', *Patient Focus Newsletter*, March 2003. London: Department of Health.

DOH (2003f) '"No NHS hospital left behind", in campaign to raise standards: every hospital fit for NHS foundation status in 4–5 years', press release 2003/0181, 6 May 2003. London: Department of Health.

DOH (2003g) *Modernisation Board – Annual Report 2002–2003*. London: Department of Health.

DOH (2003h) *Strengthening Accountability: Involving Patients and the Public*. London: Department of Health.

DOH (2003i) *Modernising Pay and Contractual Conditions for NHS Chief Executives and Directors*, consultation paper, 14 August 2003. London: Department of Health.

DOH (2003j) 'The New Medical Services Contract: what it means to Primary Care Trusts', letter to Primary Care Trust Chief Executives, 23 June 2003. London: Department of Health.

DOH (2003k) *Reimbursement: The Timing of Issuing Notices*. London: Department of Health.

DOH (2003l) *Building on the Best. Choice Responsiveness and Equity in the NHS*. London: Department of Health.

DOH (2003m) *Payment by Results, Preparing for 2005*. London: Department of Health.

DOH (2004a) *The Future Direction of the NHS Modernisation Agency*, Chief Executive Bulletin, March 2004. London: Department of Health.

DOH (2004b) *Standards for Better Health. Health Care Standards for Services under the NHS*, consultation paper, February 2004. London: Department of Health.

DOH/HM Treasury (2002). *Trackling Inequalities in Health Summary of the Cross Cutting Review 2002*. London: Department of Health.

Donaldson, L. (2003) Speech by Sir Liam Donaldson, speaking at the launch of the patient safety domain (www.'QualityHealthCare.org), 18 March 2003. London: National Patient Safety Agency.

Donnelly, L. (2003) 'Kennedy pushes for intelligent scrutiny', *Health Service Journal*, 113 (5861): 5.

Duncan Smith, I.D. (2002) *Time for Real Reform*, Conservative Party Press Conference, 9 July 2002. London: Conservative Party Headquarters.

Duncan Smith, I.D. (2003) 'Fighting for a fair deal for everybody', speech to the Conservative Party Conference, Blackpool, 9 October 2003.

Ellis, R. (ed.) (1988) 'Competence in the caring professions', in *Professional Competence and Quality Assurance in the Caring Professions*. London: Croom Helm.

Emmerson, C., Frayne, C. and Goodman, A. (2002) *How Much Would it Cost to Increase UK Health Spending to the European Average?* London: Institute for Fiscal Studies.

Enthoven, A.C. (1985) *Reflections on the Management of the National Health Service*. London: Nuffield Provincial Hospitals Trust.

Enthoven, A. (1991) 'Internal market reform of the British National Health Service', *Health Affairs*, 10 (3): 60–70.

Enthoven, A.C. (1999) *In Pursuit of Improving the National Health Service*. London: Nuffield Hospital Trust.

Eysenbach, G. and Kohler, C. (2002) 'How do consumers search for and appreciate health information on the world wide web?', *British Medical Journal*, 324: 573–7.

Florin, D. and Dixon, J. (2004) 'Public involvement in health care', *British Medical Journal*, 325 (7432): 159–61.

Flynn, R. (1992) *Structures of Control in Health Management*. London: Routledge.

Foot, M. (1999) *Aneurin Bevan 1887–1960*. London: Orion.

Fox, L. (2002) 'Focus on boosting private health care', speech to 'Civitas', Institute for Civil Society, London, 24 September 2002.

Fry, M. (ed.) (1992) *Adam Smith's Legacy*. London: Routledge.

Garside, P. and Black, A. (2003) 'Doctors in chambers', *British Medical Journal*, 326 (7390): 611–12.

Giddens, A. (1998) *The Third Way: The Renewal of Social Democracy*. Cambridge: Polity Press.

Gray, D. and Finlayson, B. (2002) 'Strong medicine', *Guardian*, 8 October 2002.

Ham, C. (1999) 'The third way in health care reform', *Journal of Health Service Research Policy*, 4 (3): 168–73.

Harman, H. (1996) *The Road to the Manifesto. Cut the Waste. Cut the Waiting*. Labour Party, London, July 1996.

Harrison, A. (2001) *Developing the Public Role in a Mixed Economy*. London: Kings Fund.

Harrison, S. and Ahmad, W. (2000) 'Medical autonomy in the UK state 1975 to 2025', *Sociology*, 34: 129–46.

Harrison, S. and Lim, J. (2003) 'The frontiers of control: doctors and managers in the NHS 1966–1997', *Clinical Governance: An International Journal*, 8 (1): 13–18.

Harrison, S., Hunter, D., Marnoch, G. and Polit, C. (1992) *Just Managing: Power and Culture in the NHS*. London: Macmillan.

HCPAC (2003a) 'Public Administration Select Committee calls for review of public service targets – and a new performance audit of government', press notice no. 16. London: House of Commons Public Administration Select Committee.

HCPAC (2003b) *Ensuring the Effective Discharge of Older Patients from Acute Hospitals*. House of Commons Public Accounts Committee. Thirty-third report of session 2002–03, HC 459. London: Stationery Office.

Health Select Committee (2003) *Foundation Trusts. Report of the All Party Health Select Committee*, 6 May 2003. London: United Kingdom Parliament.

Health Service Ombudsman (2003) *Health Service Ombudsman Selected Investigations Completed April to September 2003*, 17 December 2003. London: Office of the Health Service Ombudsman.

Higgins, R. (1993) 'Citizenship and user involvement in health provision', *Senior Nurse*, 13 (4): 14–16.

HMSO (1942) *Social Insurance and Allied Services*, Cmnd 6404. London: His Majesty's Stationery Office.

HM Treasury (2001) *Securing our Future Health: Taking a Long-Term View. Interim Report*, November 2001, by Derek Wanless. London: HM Treasury.

HM Treasury (2002a) *Securing Our Future Health: Taking a Long-Term View*. Final Report of the Health Trends Review Team, prepared by Derek Wanless. London: HM Treasury.

HM Treasury (2002b) *Budget Report 2002*. London: HM Treasury.

HM Treasury (2003) *Securing Good Health for the Whole Population: Population Health Trends*. Interim Report by Derek Wanless, December 2003. London: Stationery Office.

Hunt, S. and Symonds, S. (1995) *The Social Meaning of Midwifery*. Basingstoke: Macmillan.

Hunter, D. (2002) *Who Makes Health Policy and How?* Briefing note no. 45. London: Nuffield Trust.

IHA (2002) 'IHA calls for an end', Press release, 11 December 2002. London: Independent Health Care Association.

IPPR (2001) *Building Better Partnerships*, Final Report of the Commission on Public–Private Partnerships. London: Institute for Public Policy Research.

IPPR (2002) '*Ten myths about the PFI*', press release, 27 September 2002. London: Institute for Public Policy Research.

Johnson, J. (2004) 'BMA comments on review of star ratings: standards for better health', press release issued by the BMA chairman, 10 February 2004. London: British Medical Association.

Johnson, N. (1991) 'The break up of consensus politics in a declining economy', in M. Loney (ed.), *The State or the Market – Politics and Welfare in Contemporary Britain*, 2nd edn. London: Sage, in association with the Open University.

Kennedy, I. (2004) 'Some thoughts on CHAI's approach to scrutiny', Inaugural Annual Lecture of the Centre for Public Scrutiny, Church House, Westminster, London, 27 January 2004.

Keynes, J.M. (1973) *The Collected Writings of John Maynard Keynes*. London: Macmillan, for the Royal Economic Society.

Kings Fund (2002) *The Future NHS. A Framework for Debate*. London: Kings Fund.

Klein, R. (1995) *The New Politics of the NHS*. London: Longman.

Klein, R. (1998) 'Why Britain is reorganising its National Health Service – yet again', *Health Affairs*, 17 (4): 111–12.

Klein, R. (2001) 'Estimating the financial requirements of health care', *British Medical Journal*, 323 (7325): 1318.

Klein, R. (2003) 'Governance for NHS foundation trusts: Mr Milburn's flawed model is a cacophony of accountabilities', *British Medical Journal*, 326 (7382): 174–5.

Kmietowicz, Z. (2002) 'Government's plan for foundation hospitals comes under attack', *British Medical Journal*, 325 (7374): 1191.

Kmietowicz, Z. (2003a) 'Star rating system fails to reduce variation', *British Medical Journal*, 327 (7408): 184.

Kmietowicz, Z. (2003b) 'Foundation trusts will pressure regulator to change licence', *British Medical Journal*, 327 (7415): 581.

Labour Party (2001) *Ambitions for Britain – 2001 Manifesto*. London: Labour Party.

Lamont, S. (1999) 'Participation cannot guarantee empowerment', *British Medical Journal*, 319 (7212): 783.

Larkin, G. (1984) *Occupational Monopoly and the Profession of Medicine*. London: Tavistock.

Leatherman, S. (2003) *The Quest for Quality in the NHS*. London: Nuffield Trust.

Lewis, R. and Dixon, J. (2004) 'Rethinking chronic disease management', *British Medical Journal*, 328 (7433): 220–2.

Loney, M. (1987) *The Politics of Greed – The New Right and the Welfare State*. London: Pluto.

Marsland, D. (1994) 'Liberating welfare', in M. Pirie and D. Marsland (eds), *The End of the Welfare State*. London: Adam Smith Institute.

Marwick, C. (2003) 'Lack of health insurance costs up to $130bn in illness and premature death', *British Medical Journal*, 326 (7404): 148.

Masich, G. (1983) *Monetarism, Theory and Policy*. New York: Praeger.

McQueen, D. (2002) 'The discomfort of patient power', *British Medical Journal*, 324 (7347): 1214.

Milburn, A. (2003) 'Choice for all', speech by the Rt Hon. Alan Milburn MP, Secretary of State, to NHS chief executives, 11 February 2003.

Mintzberg, H., Ahlstrand, B. and Lampel, J. (1998) *The Strategy Safari*. New York: The Free Press.

Mooney, H. (2004) 'Tories call for Ombudsman to probe star ratings', *Health Service Journal*, 114 (5888): 4–5.

Moore, W. (2002) 'Wanless report outlines "Rolls-Royce" health service for 2022', *British Medical Journal*, 324 (7344): 998.

Morris, R. (2003) 'Passionate about the NHS', *NHS Magazine*, October 2003. Leeds: National Health Service Communications Directorate.

NAO (2003a) *NHS (England) Summarised Accounts 2001–2002*. London: National Audit Office.

NAO (2003b) *Achieving Improvement through Clinical Governance*. A progress report on implementation by NHS trusts. Report of the Comptroller General, National Audit Office, HC 1055 Session 2002–2003, 17 September 2003. London: Stationery Office.

National Centre for Social Research (2003) *British Social Attitude Survey 2003*, December 2003, London: National Centre for Social Research.

Neuberger, J. (1999) 'The NHS as a theological institution', *British Medical Journal*, 319 (7225): 1588–9.

NCSC (2003) *Protecting People and Improving Lives*. London: National Care Standards Commission.

NHS Confederation (2003) *Re-reviewing the Reviewers: The NHS Confederation's Second Survey of NHS Trust Experience of CHI Clinical Governance*. London: NHS Confederation.

NHS Executive (1998) *A First Class Service – Consultation on Quality in the New NHS*, HSC 1998/113, 1 July 1998. Leeds: National Health Service Executive.

NHS Executive (1999) *A First Class Service: Quality in the New NHS*. Leeds: NHS Executive.

OECD (2003) *Gross Domestic Product (GDP)*, National Accounts of OECD Countries, Vol. 1. Paris: Organisation of Economic Cooperation and Development.

ONS (2002) *Households covered by Medical Insurance by Socio-economic Head of Household 1998–1999*, Social Trends 30. London: Office of National Statistics.

ONS (2003) *Economic Trends No. 592*. London: Office of National Statistics (also at www.statistics.gov.uk).

Pariera, J. (1989) 'What does equity in health mean?', Discussion Paper No. 61, Centre for Health Economics, University of York.

Pietroni, P., Winkler, F. and Graham, L. (2003) 'Cultural revolution', *British Medical Journal*, 326 (7404): 1304–6.

Pirie, M. and Worcester, R.M. (2001) *The Wrong Package*. London: Adam Smith Institute.

Plsek, P.E. and Greenhalgh, T. (2001) 'The challenge of complexity in health care', *British Medical Journal*, 323 (7313): 625–8.

Plsek, P.E. and Wilson, T. (2001) 'Complexity, leadership and management in healthcare organisations', *British Medical Journal*, 323 (7315): 746–9.

Plumridge, N. (2003) 'Going with the flow', *Health Service Journal*, 113 (5867): 31.

Pollit, C., Birchall, J. and Putnam, K. (1997) *Decentralising Public Service Management*. London: Macmillan.

Pollock, A. (2003) 'Foundation hospitals will kill the NHS. Don't be fooled by the rhetoric', *The Guardian*, 7 May 2003.

Pollock, A., Shaoul, J., Rowland, D. and Player, S. (2001) *Public Services and the Private Sector*. London: Catalyst.

Pollock, A., Shaoul, J. and Vickers, N. (2002) 'Private finance and value for money in NHS hospitals: a policy in search of a rationale', *British Medical Journal*, 324 (7345): 1205–9.

Powell, M. (2000) 'Analysing the "new" British National Health Service', *International Journal of Health Planning and Management*, 15: 89–101.

Reform (2003) *A Better Way*, Commission on the Reform of Public Services. London: Reform.

Reid, J. (2003) 'More choice, more fairness in the NHS', speech by Health Secretary Dr John Reid, Secretary of State for Health, to the AMICUS conference, Whitehall College, Bishop's Stortford, 17 September 2003.

Robinson, R. (2002) 'NHS foundation trusts: greater autonomy may prove illusory', *British Medical Journal*, 325 (7363): 506–7.

Rowland, D.R. and Pollock, A.M. (2004) 'Choice and responsiveness for older people in the "patient centred" NHS', *British Medical Journal*, 328 (7430): 4–5.

Royal Statistical Society (2003) *Performance Indicators: Good, Bad and Ugly*. London: Royal Statistical Society.

Sassi, R., Archard, L. and Le Grand, J. (2001) 'Equity versus efficiency: a dilemma for the NHS', *British Medical Journal*, 323 (7316): 762.

Say, R.E. and Thomson, R. (2003) 'The importance of patient preferences in treatment decisions – the challenge for doctors', *British Medical Journal*, 327 (7414): 542–5.

Scally, G. and Donaldson, L.J. (1998) 'Clinical governance and the drive for quality improvement in the new NHS in England', *British Medical Journal*, 317 (7150): 61–5.

Sergeant, H. (2003) *Managing not to Manage. The Story of Failure at the Heart of British Hospitals*. London: Centre for Policy Studies.

Slevin, M. (2003) *Resuscitating the NHS – A Consultant's View*. London: Centre for Policy Studies.

Smith, P. (2003) 'A and E awaits a single week of judgement', *Health Service Journal*, 113 (5847): 6–7.

Smith, R. (2003a) 'Changing the leadership of the NHS', *British Medical Journal*, 326 (7403): 1.

Smith, R. (2003b) 'What doctors and managers can learn from each other', *British Medical Journal*, 326 (7370): 610–11.

Spiers, J. (1995) *The Invisible Hospital and Secret Garden*. Oxford: Radcliffe Medical Press.

Stationery Office (2001a) Public inquiry into children's heart surgery in Bristol 1984–1995', in *Learning from Bristol*. London: Stationery Office.

Stationery Office (2001b) *Report of the Comptroller and Auditor General – Managing the Relationship to Secure a Successful Partnership in PFI Projects*. London: Stationery Office.

Stationery Office (2002) *Health Select Committee. First Report of Session 2001–02 (HC 308) Inquiry into the Role of the Private Sector in the NHS*. London: Stationery Office.

Stewart, M. (1993) *Keynes in the 1990s, a Return to Economic Sanity*. London: Penguin.

Timmins, N. (1996) *The Five Giants – A Biography of the Welfare State*. London: HarperCollins.

Titmuss, R.M. and Morris, R. (1973) *Social Policy, an Introduction*. London: Allen & Unwin.

Titmuss, R.M. and Morris, R. (1976) *Essays on the Welfare State*. London: Allen & Unwin.

Towse, A. and Sussex, J. (2000) 'Getting UK health care up to the European Union "mean": what does that mean?', *British Medical Journal*, 320 (7235): 640–2.

UNISON (2003) 'Gives MPs 7 reasons to oppose foundation hospitals', press release, 31 March 2003, London.

UNISON (2004) 'Private companies stitch up NHS', press release, 5 February 2004, London.

Walshe, K. (2003) 'New structures of governance needed', *British Medical Journal*, 326 (7392): 764–5.

Warden, J. (1998) 'Britain's new welfare system emphasises self-reliance', *British Medical Journal*, 316 (7137): 1037.

Wardrope, J. (2002) 'Unlimited consumer demand would destroy the NHS', *British Medical Journal*, 322 (7298): 1369.

Warner, M., Longley, M., Gould, E. and Picek, A. (1998) *Health Futures 2010. Welsh Institute for Health and Social Care*. Pontypridd: University of Glamorgan.

Whitehead, M. (1994) 'Who cares about equity in the NHS?', *British Medical Journal*, 308: 1284–7.

WHO (1998) *Health Promotion Glossary*. Geneva World Health Organisation.

Wilkins, R. (2000) 'Poor relations: the paucity of the professional paradigm', in M. Kirkham (ed.), *The Midwife–Mother Relationship*. London: Macmillan.

Wilkinson, P. (2003) 'Under new management', *NHS Magazine*, March 2003, pp. 14–15.

Wilmot, S. (2003) *Ethics Power and Policy. The Future of Nursing in the NHS*. Basingstoke: Palgrave.

Yoong, K.Y. and Heyman, T. (2003) 'Target centred medicine. Targets can seriously damage your health', *British Medical Journal*, 327 (7416): 680.

INDEX

Compiled by INDEXING SPECIALISTS (UK)
LIMITED, 202 Church Road, Hove, East
Sussex BN3 2DJ. Tel: 01273 738299.
Email: richardr@indexing.co.uk Website:
www.indexing.co.uk